Your 10 Step™ Ey
Action Plan

(A 3-month to 12-month action plan to recover your Eyesight Health.)

By Robert Redfern

To help with:

- ❖ Macular Degeneration (Wet and Dry)
- ❖ Glaucoma
- ❖ Computer Eye Strain Syndrome
- ❖ Conjunctivitis
- ❖ Cataracts
- ❖ Diabetic Retinopathy
- ❖ Hereditary (Genetic) - Retinitis Pigmentosa, Juvenile Macular Degeneration.
- ❖ Multiple Sclerosis (MS) eye problems
- ❖ Dry Eye / Blepharitis
- ❖ Common Eye Problems (near sighted, far sighted etc.)

using safe, natural remedies pioneered by doctors in the USA.

Phone enquiries 0800 015 1580
Eye queries — David. (Ext 3)

This book is dedicated...

...to those doctors who have stuck their head above the parapet, who went against the "norm" in their "group thinking," and who helped find successful solutions to common degenerative diseases. Such doctors give people the independence and quality of life they were told would come in the 21st century. To all those who strive for breakthrough and excellence in the utilization of natural remedies that vitally enhance our health and well-being, I salute you.

These include:

Julian Kenyon, M.D. (UK)
Robert O. Becker, M.D. (USA)
Bjorn Nordenstrom, M.D. (Sweden)
Grace Halloran, Ph.D. (USA)
Edward C. Kondrot, M.D. (USA)
Jonathan Wright, M.D. (USA)
Robert O. Young, Ph.D. (USA)
Gary Price Todd, Ophthalmologist (USA)
Stanley Evans (UK and Africa)
Peter Mansfield, M.D. (UK)
Professor James Philips, Chairman, International Obesity Task Force

This list comprises but a few names of the thousands of doctors and natural health practitioners around the world who have successfully treated eye diseases for many years, utilizing natural methods with great success, including proper nutrition and MicroCurrent stimulation.

There is another group of doctors and natural health practitioners who also found that cleansing the body, restoring the digestive system back to health, and applying proper nutrition helps the vast majority of people be restored to good health. Other interventions, such as acupuncture, homeopathy, and herbs have also been used with great success.

This book is also dedicated to the doctors, some of which were awarded the Nobel Prize for their work, who have proven scientifically the various solutions discussed in this book.

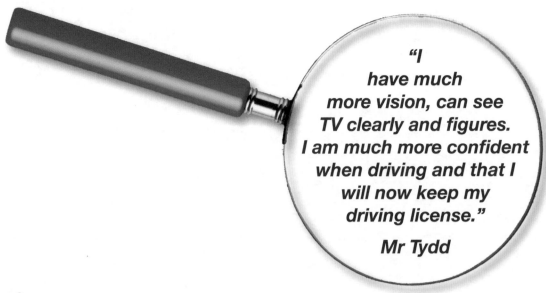

"I have much more vision, can see TV clearly and figures. I am much more confident when driving and that I will now keep my driving license."

Mr Tydd

> *"My eyes are now marvelous; the Lutein spray has improved my eyes tremendously. I am surprised the doctors do not prescribe it."*
>
> *Mrs. Campbell*

What you may not know about your so-called "balanced diet"

Nutritionist Dr. David Thomas, gave the following findings on mineral depletion at a lecture (published in the Nutrition & Health, Journal of the McCarrison Society for Nutrition & Health, Vol. 17:no. 2, 2003):

Between 1940 and 1991...

Vegetables were depleted of:	Fruits were depleted of:
76% of their copper	19% of their copper
49% of their sodium	9% of their sodium
46% of their calcium	16% of their calcium
27% of their iron	24% of their iron
24% of their magnesium	15% of their magnesium
16% of their potassium	22% of their potassium

The importance of the facts listed above relates to the nutrition and supplementation of nutrients that are vital to your 10 Step™ Eye Health Action Plan. Without proper nutrition, all of your body's organs are affected, leading to many of our modern day sicknesses and diseases.

We will also discuss not only the need for nutritional supplements in your diet, as part of your recommended healthy lifestyle changes, but also the importance of absorbing those nutrients.

Part 1 – Overview and FAQs

Overview

There are many established natural therapies for the health of your eyes. By reading these pages, you will discover:

    a. Which eye diseases are helped with the 10 Step™ Eye Health Plan

    b. Why you are only now discovering such remedies

    c. How it is possible to improve the health of your eyes

    d. How you can plan for the future health of your eyes

You cannot be guaranteed 100% recovery from any condition, but if you do nothing, you are guaranteed your condition could get worse or, at best, stay as it is.

I have spoken to thousands of sufferers of various eye problems, and all have articulated their passion to empower themselves to recover the health of their eyes. Therefore, this book is written as a 10 Step™ plan to enable you to have the best chance of recovering your eye health. NOTE: It may take 3-12 months to achieve your best possible recovery.

The 10 Step™ plan does not simply involve popping a pill. For some of you, it may involve making difficult lifestyle changes. The more steps you take, the better your chances of recovery. I have not spoken to anyone who is unwilling to take these necessary steps to recover their sight, as the ability to see is so vital to their quality of everyday life.

You may get upset, as others have, when you learn that these simple therapies have been known for many years, and particularly, when you realize that the earlier they are put to use, the greater your chance of a successful outcome.

This book makes no attempt to explain scientifically how it all works. It is simply common nutritional/biological sense that is explained. Nevertheless, everything in this book is based upon the simple fact that doctors in the USA are using these steps on their patients, with a 70%-80% success rate, either in stopping the diseases or in reversing them.

Age-Related Macular Degeneration (ARMD) has much the same origins as most of the diseases that afflict us today, i.e., nutritional deficiency of some kind. Scurvy, rickets, beriberi, heart disease, and now even cancer have all been shown to be diseases directly related to problems in diet and nutrition.

This is a book for the millions of people who have been previously condemned to a dark future, and who now have an opportunity to see the light, both metaphorically and literally. To realize this opportunity, you will need to apply the actions outlined in this book for 3-12 months, and/ or until you have gained a substantial improvement in your eyesight. After that time, you will need to continue a maintenance program throughout your life to ensure you never lose your eyesight again.

Frequently Asked Questions

What is ARMD?

Age-Related Macular Degeneration (ARMD) is a condition that can normally affect you as you age. In fact, though it is the leading cause of sight loss in those over 50 years of age, it is now appearing in individuals as young as 20 years of age. Essentially, ARMD is caused by the huge amount of free radical damage inflicted by sunlight, poor nutrition, toxins, and the lack of nutrients reaching the macula to protect it from this free radical damage. The two specific nutrients responsible for protecting the macula are Lutein (loo-teen) and Zeaxanthin (zeeah-zan-thin). These carotenoids are powerful antioxidants that are known to be reduced in the eyes of ARMD sufferers (see page 41).

ARMD affects the macula, which is the small part of the eye responsible for central vision, and which allows you to see detail and colors. ARMD usually starts in one eye and is then highly likely to affect the other at a later stage.

"Wet" and "Dry" ARMD

Dry ARMD is the most common form of the condition, and it usually develops slowly, until eventually, it leads to a loss of up to 95% of central vision. Depending upon its severity, this form of ARMD is relatively easy to stop and reverse, with simple changes in nutrition and lifestyle. Dry ARMD occurs when the buildup of waste material is no longer cleared from the macula, and there is a lack of nutrients reaching the eyes.

Wet ARMD is caused by weak and undernourished blood vessels that grow behind the retina and leak into the macula. It is less common than the dry form of ARMD, but it can cause a more rapid vision loss.

What causes ARMD (and other eye diseases)?

While the majority of mainstream orthodox doctors are still baffled as to its cause, the majority of natural health practitioners are now confident of the following causes, which include:

1. Poor diet (not enough greens and healthy fats, or simply eating the wrong foods)
2. Lack of nutrients in the diet (over farming, factory processing, and natural erosion have led to severe mineral deficiency in foods)
3. Food intolerances, causing poor nutrient absorption (shown in the majority of cases by general or severe digestive problems)
4. Genetic predisposition and nutritional absorption problems (usually considered hereditary, perhaps instead due to poor nutritional habits learned in families)
5. Smoking and other toxic overloads, such as drugs, alcohol, saturated fats, etc.
6. Generally, those who suffer poor health, as a result of nutritional problems, will eventually suffer some form of eye disease, as in the case of diabetics
7. Arteriosclerosis
8. Sex/genes
9. Iris color

Cross section through the eye

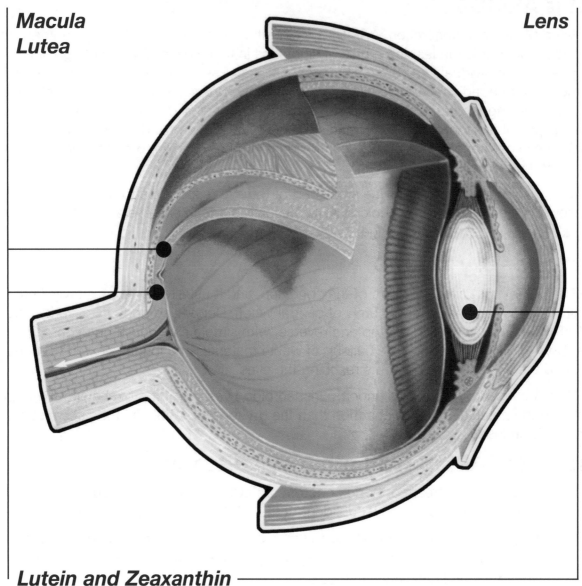

Macula Lutea

Lens

Lutein and Zeaxanthin
(The largest concentration in the body is found in these two places)

How common is ARMD?

It has been estimated that over 25% of the population over the age of 65 will suffer some form of sight loss. That does not include the frightening prospect of the younger generation, who are already showing signs as young as only 20 years of age. The positive news is that only one in seven of those sufferers will develop the wet form of ARMD.

With the prospect of many millions of the population suffering some form of sight loss, a major crisis is looming, unless the public is informed of the causes—and solutions—mentioned herein.

The chance of developing ARMD increases as you get older, unless you either change or improve upon your nutritional and lifestyle habits. Even then, no one can guarantee 100% success, but the majority of those who suffer can save their sight or radically improve it.

The following pages show you the symptoms of ARMD, as well as simple tests you can do to measure its early symptoms. Other eye diseases are also discussed, with suggestions and solutions recommended for recovery for each in the pages to follow.

How does ARMD affect vision?

ARMD affects different people in different ways and, in its early stages, you may notice changes in your vision, such as:

❖ Blurred vision with close work

❖ Seeing straight lines as wavy (doorways may appear as a figure 8)

❖ Your sight degrades as you look straight at print or at faces

❖ A black hole, which starts grey and goes steadily blacker, may form in the center of your vision

❖ Sensitivity to bright light accompanied by poor night vision

❖ You can only adapt from light to dark very slowly

❖ Eventually, you may only have a small amount of peripheral vision

You will need to have a consultation with a good eye doctor to identify precisely what is wrong. However, since many optometrists or ophthalmologists are unaware of the many breakthroughs in nutrition regarding eyesight recovery, they may not believe anything can be done. If this is the case, it may be best to take your eye health into your own hands. But you will not be alone. Eyesight Action will help you through the process of your eye health recovery with our easy-to-follow 10 Step™ Eye Health Recovery Plan.

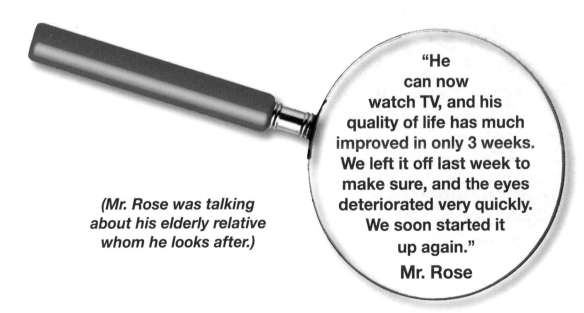

(Mr. Rose was talking about his elderly relative whom he looks after.)

"He can now watch TV, and his quality of life has much improved in only 3 weeks. We left it off last week to make sure, and the eyes deteriorated very quickly. We soon started it up again."
Mr. Rose

The visual effects of ARMD...

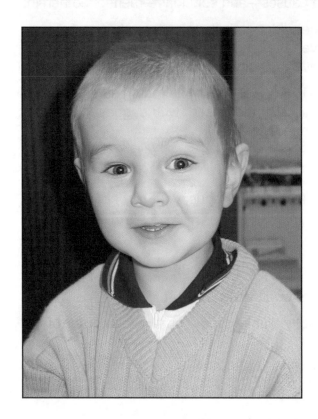

Normal Vision

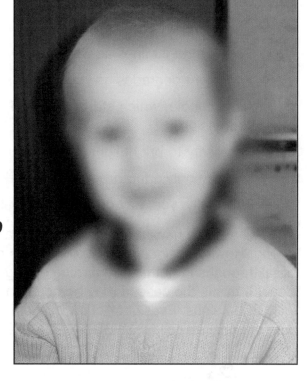

Early ARMD

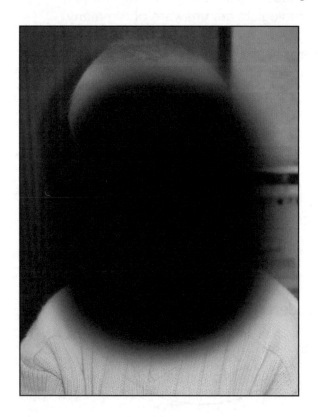

Advanced ARMD

Testing for early symptoms of ARMD

The Amsler Grid

The Amsler grid was originally developed by Marc Amsler to allow patients to test their own central vision for early signs of macular degeneration. This test consists of a grid of vertical and horizontal lines.

Directions:

- Look through your reading glasses or bifocals.

- Cover the left eye. While looking at the centre dot from a distance of 12 inches or so, answer the following questions: Can you see all four corners of the grid? Are any of the lines blurry, wavy, distorted, bent, grey, or missing?

- Repeat the previous step, this time covering the right eye.

If you note any changes in how you see the grid, call your eye doctor for evaluation.

We recommend that you keep the grid where you can use it 2-3 times a week.

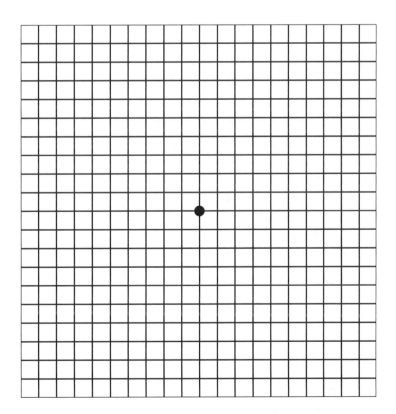

Use the Amsler grid, as well as the chart on the following page, to plot your recovery progress with your action plan.

Points		Optitypes	Power	Diopters
72		N L Z		48
48		H N L E	8.0	32
36		T Z N H F	6.5	26
26		Z F N T L H	5.0	20
20		E N H L Z T	3.5	14
16		L E Z T N F	3.0	12
14		F T Z H N L	2.5	10
12		L H T N F Z	2.0	8
10		T L E Z H N	1.7	7
9		F T N E L H	1.5	6
8		Z H E N T F	1.0	4

Points			Power	Diopters
		Optitypes	**Pure Focus**	**Supplied By**
Date	Data	**Optigram Directions**		
		Start at 72, work your way down until the number reading slows. Then read the letters to the right. Repeat once a week or as directed.	Take 2 pumps under the tongue, 3 to 5 times a day or as directed	If you need help, call the Helpline, shown at the front of the book

What to do next if your test does not look normal

If you think you may be experiencing symptoms of ARMD (or any other eye problem) you need to make an action plan.

1. Consider a consultation with an eye professional.
2. Consider the probable causes on page 5, and rectify any lifestyle shortcomings.
3. As a minimum, start your recovery plan by improving your diet.
4. Follow the full 10 Step™ Plan on page 17 and the subsequent pages.
5. If you need help, call the Helpline, shown at the front of the book.

Other nutrition related conditions that affect the eyes are:

❖ Cataracts

❖ Glaucoma

❖ Diabetic Retinopathy

❖ Dry Eyes

❖ Computer Eye Syndrome

❖ Failing Eyesight

❖ Myopathy

❖ Retinitis Pigmentosa

Eyesight Professionals

Dispensing Opticians are not qualified to diagnose eyesight problems.
Dispensing opticians are specially trained to take essential measurements to enable the manufacture of glasses, according to the prescription from an optometrist. They also make sure the glasses fit properly and advise on style and shape. With further training, they can fit contact lenses.

An Ophthalmologist is qualified to diagnose and treat all eye conditions.
Ophthalmologists are medically qualified surgeons, specializing in eye disease and treatment, and carry out eye operations when necessary. Unfortunately, they do not have any training in nutrition and, therefore, may not appreciate the new studies showing that many eye conditions can be stopped and reversed. Unless they have studied nutrition and taken a great interest in the new studies, there may not be any benefit in asking for their advice with regard to nutritional effects upon eyesight recovery.

Optometrists examine and test eyes for diseases and defects.
Optometrists can also give advice for general health and lifestyle problems appertaining to defects in eyesight. In a clinical setting, they advise on corrective options, prescribe glasses and contact lenses, issue (subject to current studies) nutritional and health care advice, monitor eye conditions, and refer eye disorders that, ultimately, cannot be managed in a primary care (non-hospital) setting to ophthalmologists.

Our advice is to find an optometrist or ophthalmologist who is prepared to look at the overwhelming data showing that poor nutrition and lifestyle are the cause of the majority of eye diseases, which can be greatly improved through proper nutrition and lifestyle changes.

Typical Questions

What about conditions other than Macular Degeneration?

The specific actions are detailed with the exact program for each eye problem in the Appendix.

What causes this deterioration to happen?

Orthodox eye doctors are not required to have training in nutrition and, consequently, may tell you there are no known causes of eyesight-related conditions. We concur with a different group of doctors, with expert knowledge in the field of nutrition, who have found that it is contributed to significantly, or exacerbated by, malnutrition or nutritional deficiencies. We need the following to sustain vibrant life and health every day:

- ❖ Proteins, fats, carbohydrates.
- ❖ 13 or so vitamins
- ❖ 20-60 minerals (the number depends which scientists you believe)
- ❖ 12 or so amino acids
- ❖ 10 or so essential fatty acids
- ❖ 6 or so digestive enzymes (from plants)
- ❖ Oxygen
- ❖ Pure Water (such as distilled, bottled, or purified tap water)
- ❖ Probiotics (the healthy bacteria that should be in your intestines)

All of the listed factors need to be in place, as they all work interactively or as cofactors to each other, and any deficiency will result in a malfunction. For example, there are over 80 enzymes at work in your body that need zinc as a cofactor.

Rarely are all these essential nutrients found in our daily diet, even if you were certain your digestive system were absorbing them all. Are you absorbing your nutrition? Absorption is key, as you will come to understand, as I explain, as clearly as possible, what may go wrong with your eyes due to lack of nutrition.

You need many specific antioxidants to counteract the free-radical damage that results from your body's energy creation. Free radicals are caused by sunlight acting upon our eyes, and by cellular combustion when we generate energy, as well as elevated levels of glucose in our bloodstream. We should have two specific antioxidants in our eyes, Lutein (lu-teen) and Zeaxanthin (zee-a-zan-than). Antioxidants help to counter this free radical activity (see studies in the Appendix). We can, therefore, conclude that it is necessary to have an abundance of these nutrients in our eyes.

Why do we not have them? Let us look at the antioxidants Lutein and Zeaxanthin. These are found in abundance in dark leafy green vegetables. There are five reasons why you may be lacking these nutrients in the eye:

1. You simply may not eat enough dark leafy green nutrient-rich vegetables each day. A list of vegetables and their content is shown later.

2. As we get older, we do not absorb food from our digestive system as well as we did when we were younger. This is mainly caused by a lack of HCL (acid) in the stomach and a lack of digestive enzymes in the food. A study shows that the average 70-year-old has only 20% of the beneficial enzymes available compared to a 20-year-old. This is caused mainly by overeating enzymatically dead foods. There is an urgent need to increase enzyme intake, either by way of the food we eat, or by taking supplements to help make up for this poor absorption. For example, a small glass of apple cider vinegar just before each meal will stimulate stomach acid.

3. Food intolerance to wheat or dairy products is very common. This blocks the uptake of nutrients in the digestive tract. If you have this problem, you probably already suffer digestive problems, such as indigestion, acid reflux, and bowel diseases, such as Crohn's Disease, piles, colitis, IBS, etc. (This intolerance can also have a genetic factor)

4. Eating too many grains, cereals, and dairy products can replace or block proper nutrition. Wheat, grains, and dairy products are not appropriate nutrition for good health. The negative aspect of these foods is amplified by the processes they endure before they reach our grocery shelves and by the depletion of even more nutrients during storage and food preparation.

5. As a result of an inappropriate diet, the blood stream can suffer clogging, as described in No. 4 above. Poor absorption and smoking (studies show smokers are 2.5 times more likely to get eye disease), causes the tiny veins in the eye to be blocked, thereby starving your eye of essential nutrients.

ATP is a nutrient produced in your own cells for all of your energy needs. Your body needs the equivalent of your own body weight of ATP every day, to supply its energy needs. To produce this, your cells (as well as essential fatty acids) need to absorb oxygen and glucose in a ratio of 80% to 20% for the huge amount of ATP needed. This ATP is essential, as discussed earlier, not only for your body's physical energy but also for cell cleaning and cell regeneration. Unfortunately, this process causes damaging, combustive, free radical activity (oxidation). These free radicals damage the healthy cells and can only be stopped by eating a good amount of fruit and vegetables with their powerful supply of antioxidants. The antioxidants Lutein and Zeaxanthin are the specific antioxidants that alleviate this free radical activity in the eyes and are, therefore, vital for the healthy aging of your eyes (and the rest of your body).

Premature aging and degeneration is believed by many researchers to be caused in part by a deficiency of ATP. The delicate ratio (80% Oxygen : 20% Glucose) balance can easily be upset by too much glucose from eating starchy foods. Combining this with a deficiency of oxygen from poor breathing or insufficient aerobic exercising can cause an ATP deficiency. When this happens, our cells reduce their output of ATP and produce a toxic substance called Lactic Acid.

An ATP deficiency will result in a loss of energy which may influence you to reduce your normal amount of exercise. To make matters worse, you may also mistakenly take in more sugars and starchy foods in an effort to gain more energy, thereby poisoning your cells' regeneration even more. Another way that glucose damages our cells is by means of "glycated proteins," which produce 50 times more free radicals than non glycated proteins. Research indicates Glycation may also be a prime factor in cataracts, brain disease, and other health problems. Any lack of antioxidants and ATP will inhibit your cells' ability to regenerate, thereby causing overall premature aging and DAMAGE TO YOUR EYES.

Anti-Ageing Theory—There are good studies conducted on animals in the laboratory, showing that by greatly reducing the level of calories in foods they ate, the life expectancy of animals doubled, compared to those eating high calorie foods (the biggest culprits of which are grains, cereals, potatoes, and sugars). The animals eating low calorie foods, such as vegetables, nuts and seeds, did not suffer from age-related degenerative diseases, whereas those eating high calorie food did. Do you need any other motivation for cutting back on grains, cereals, sugars and potatoes? (See the Glycemic Index of food for balanced blood sugar foods in the Appendix.)

How long have doctors been successfully treating Eye Diseases?

Eye Diseases have been successfully treated for about ten years in the USA, and these successes have been widely reported for the past five years.. So get started on working to get your eyes healthy, then shout your results from the rooftops to help others who have suffered just like you get their recovery as well.

Why has my doctor not told me about these Therapies?

It is a cultural and training problem. I have lectured many times to doctors and found them to be uninformed about new research around the world. Their training basically tells them that nutrition is not the prime cause of degenerative diseases and therefore they will not even consider this concept as they fear it would open them up to criticism or ridicule from their peers. If you want to learn about the real manipulators, who control the health system (and spread misinformation about the benefits of nutrition) you should read books written by doctors who have exposed the anti-public activities of drug companies and medical organisations (see book list at back).

Are these therapies safe?

Yes. Essentially the 10 Steps™ will help return your eyes to healthy functioning. A by-product of this process is that your body will become healthier, too.

What are my chances of getting better?

Doctors in the USA report a 70%-80% success rate when they are working closely with their patients and giving them expert advice, especially in the early stages. There are those who have faithfully applied the 10 Steps to their daily life and nutrition and enjoyed recovery within just a few weeks. Others have taken from three to 12 months for the same results. The simple fact is, the longer you follow the 10 Steps™, and the more of them you do, the better your chances of recovery. At the very least, you can prevent your eyesight from getting any worse.

Do I have to do all 10 Steps™, and is there any special order I have to do them in?

Simply start at Step 1. The more you do, the better your chances of recovery.

Please take note:

The "10 Steps™ to Natural Eye Health" are completely safe, and we recommend you try them before considering corrective surgery (after consulting with your doctor, of course). It is worthy to note that 3% of patients that have cataract operations go on to develop complications, including infection, swelling, detachment of the retina, and glaucoma.

Success Report—the First 600 Surveyed

Lutein and MicroCurrent stimulation for the treatment of macular degeneration and other eye diseases has been popularized in the UK by the TV appearance of Dr. Chris Steele on the Richard and Judy "This Morning" program. This followed a report in the Daily Mail, outlining the good results obtained by doctors in the USA.

A telephone survey was carried out among the first 600 people who were taking Lutein spray and/or using the MicroCurrent stimulator. The following figures show the reported results of those contacted:

- ❖ 62% reported definite to good eyesight return
- ❖ 37% reported that their condition had not gotten any worse, but they could not detect an improvement.
- ❖ Less than 1% said it made no difference, and/or it had become worse.

NOTE:

- ❖ No one surveyed had any personal help or support from a qualified person and had treated themselves or were helped by a relative or friend.
- ❖ Not one person had started to use any of the additional nutrients detailed in this book.

Conclusions:

1. We believe these results confirm this program is suitable for the majority of individuals who desire to self-treat their eyes at home.
2. Those who need support will only need a minimal amount, until they get sufficient sight recovery, at which time, they can manage for themselves.

A Typical Report from the Survey

Mrs C.

> *"I can now see close-up print for the first time in ten years. I have had a substantial improvement. I have now got my husband on it and I have told all our friends".*

An exceptional Report from the Survey

Mrs T

> *"Eighteen months ago I was blind in one eye and then the other eye started to rapidly go the same way. By January this year (2001) I was effectively blind in both eyes. By then I was devastated.*
>
> *In February (I think it was this date), I heard Dr Chris Steele say on the morning television program that patients who were blind had taken a nutrient under their tongue and within a few months they were able to drive their cars again. I was very excited at this and tried to telephone the TV station but the lines were engaged. I tried for a few weeks in desperation and finally got through to get the telephone number of the distributor. I immediately called and started taking the spray under my tongue. After 3-4 months of taking it I knew things were dramatically improving, but preferred to hear what my consultant said before I got too excited. **After he examined me he said that he***

could not explain it but my eyes had grown new blood vessels and repaired themselves. *He said he had never experienced this and had only heard about it in young people. When I tried to tell him about the Lutein spray and what I had done he brushed me off and seemed not to want to listen. I was astonished that he would not want to know and recommend it to his other patients.*

A few days later I went to see my optician, eager to hear his report. **He said that he was astonished to report that my eyesight was now BETTER than 20:20, which is better than it had ever been. He was eager to hear about the Lutein Spray and was genuinely thrilled at its success***. I feel I have a future again".*

> **"I no longer need reading glasses, and I can see to do my crossword easily."**
>
> **Mrs. Marie**

> **"My-mother uses it, and she can now go to the shops on her own. We are both very happy and amazed at the results."**
>
> **Mrs Reeve**

Part 2 - 10 Step™ Eye Health Plan

Overview

1. Take Lutein spray and the other recommended nutrients beneficial to your eyes (see the detailed list contained in this book).

2. Drink 8 oz. of filtered, bottled, or boiled water 8-12 times per day (not within 30 minutes before or after eating a meal).

3. Foods to **include** in your diet are vegetables (eight portions per day). Kale, spinach, and carrots are all good selections. Eat as many different colors as possible. Fruit, nuts, seeds, beans, eggs, and fish (different types of fish 3-4 times per week) should be included as well. For recipe ideas, see the Appendix.

4. Foods to **exclude** from your diet are breads, pastries, biscuits, breakfast cereals, pasta, root vegetables (potatoes, parsnips, etc.) and others high in carbohydrates for at least three to six months.

5. Exercise every day to get oxygen around your body, your lungs working, and your heart beating faster. Walking, running in place, and rebounding on a mini-trampoline are best. Alternatively, if you are immobile, take OxySorb enzymes to improve oxygen absorption.

6. Take other enzymes and probiotics and recommend nutrients listed in this book, such as gingko, bilberry, and vitamin A.

7. Consider an herbal cleanse/detox to recover your digestive system.

8. Ask us for details of homeopathic remedies and doctors via e-mail at www.eyesight.nu.

9. If you have blocked arteries, oral chelation therapy, along with serrapeptase, the enzyme recommended for clearing arteries without the need for surgery, is recommended. (For more information, visit www.serrapeptase.info or call the help line, shown at the front of the book.)

10. Use your Microcurrent stimulator, if you have one, as per the instructions in this book. (To purchase one, go to www.goodhealthnaturally.com/ (UK) / www.goodhealthusa.com (USA) or call the help line, shown at the front of the book.)

10 Step™ Eye Health Plan - Step 1

Essential Nutrients for Healthy Eyes

a. **Lutein and Zeaxanthin** are the only two carotenoids found in the eye with the specific job of overcoming free radical damage. These critical nutrients are, therefore, essential steps for healthy eyes, as well as your lungs and heart. The form we recommend you take them in is a spray.

Why is it important to take these nutrients in spray form, rather than in tablet form? This is a very important point. Sublingual (under the tongue) delivery gives nearly 95% absorption. If you have a problem with poor digestion or absorption for any reason, nutrients in tablet form will get lost in the long passage to the eye via the digestive system. Taking these nutrients in a sublingual spray form ensures they are absorbed directly into the bloodstream in only seconds, and they are present in the eye within minutes. They are aided additionally by gingko and bilberry, which improve blood flow and the integrity of the capillaries, especially in the eyes and brain. (See the chart on page 42.)

b. **Taurine** is an amino acid found naturally in eggs and fish, as well as other foods. It is necessary for healthy eyes and act as an antioxidant. It helps gets nutrients into your cells, while also helping to remove cell debris and other potentially toxic substances from your eyes.

Why the need for taurine? As your digestive system becomes dysfunctional, your absorption of taurine diminishes. You will almost certainly need to supplement in the short-term for your eye recovery plan. You may need "friendly bacteria" to aide its absorption.

c. **Multi Vitamins, Minerals & Trace Minerals.** This is a supplement that everybody needs daily, as a result of the dramatically reduced vitamin and mineral content in your food (even if you eat fresh organic foods every day). We show you the perfect formulation in the appendix of essential vitamins, antioxidants, folic acid and over 70 ionic trace minerals. This is the most complete daily supplement, especially since it also contains the selenium you need. Numerous studies show a long list of conditions it can help, in addition to your eyes, including cancer, heart disease, immune system dysfunction, and many others (see the list of studies in the Appendix). Taking 1fl.oz. daily is sufficient to give you the vitamins and minerals needed to improve overall health

d. **Essential Fatty Acids (EFAs)** are essential daily for the health of your body, and especially for your eyes, circulatory system, and brain. EFA's are very important and healthy nutrients which are found in about 5-6 different oils. They are not all found in cod liver oil or primrose oil. They include Omega-3 and Omega-6, EPA, GLA, and DHA (from oily fish). There are two ways to nourish your body with them. One way is to buy a ready-prepared complex of fish oils that contains all of the required EFA's you need for your health. We recommend a vegetarian product called Hemp Oil, which is often called the "Master of All Oils," to ensure you get all the EFA's necessary for optimum health.

e. **Antioxidants** stop free radical damage in its tracks. We have found AstaXanthin to be the best, with 500 times the power of vitamin E.

f. **MSM+Silver Water Drops** consist of organic sulphur and colloidal silver and have a good history of aiding eye health by softening the tissue and improving the eye's ability to absorb nutrients. Silver is a natural infection killer.

Step 1—Nutrients Action Step

1. Take Lutein spray, 12 sprays per day (therapeutic dose) until you obtain definite recovery. Then take the maintenance dose of 6 sprays per day.

   a. Spray the Lutein Spray under your tongue or in your mouth 4 times upon rising.

   b. Repeat with 4 sprays mid-afternoon and again in the evening.

   c. Swish the Lutein around your mouth for about two minutes, before swallowing.

2. Take 5-8 sprays of Taurine daily (can be at the same time as Lutein).

3. Take Multi-vitamins/mineral supplement in a divided dose with breakfast and dinner.

4. Take 10 ml of Essential Fatty Acids Oil Complex with breakfast and 10ml with dinner.

5. Take an antioxidant. (Astaxanthin is highly recommended).

6. Take MSM+Silver Water Drops. (Take one drop every hour or so.)

"The consultant at the hospital told me that my macular degeneration had unusually stopped getting any worse but that it could not be anything to do with the Lutein spray. My optician however measured a definite improvement and has written to the consultant querying why they would say that Lutein would not work when obviously it has. My left eye, which was still deteriorating after laser surgery, is also improving. I can see everything in good detail now. I am re-applying for my driving license."

Mrs. Lewis

10 Step™ Eye Health Plan - Step 2

Water

Water is an essential component of maintaining life, yet many of us don't drink nearly enough. Many natural health practitioners found that a major part of the epidemic of degenerative diseases is dehydration from insufficient water consumption. You need to increase your water intake to at least 64 oz. per day. Tea, coffee, juices, and soft drinks are fluids, and do not constitute water for this purpose. If all you have is tap water, consider a good filter as the inorganic minerals and chlorine can cause problems.

Step 2—Water Actions—Look at the filter options in the data sheets in the Appendix, and decide whether one is needed for you.

1. On waking, drink 16-32 oz. of warm water (or at least room temp), and do not eat or drink anything for one hour. The purpose of this is to hydrate the colon. You may temporarily increase this to 48 oz. if you are suffering constipation.

2. About one hour after breakfast drink another 8 oz. glass, and continue to drink a glass of water every hour until 7 PM. in the evening. The total number of glasses not including your first, should be about 12.

3. It is up to you how much tea and coffee you drink.

4. Alcohol is poisonous to human bodies, so avoid it while doing the Steps, if possible.

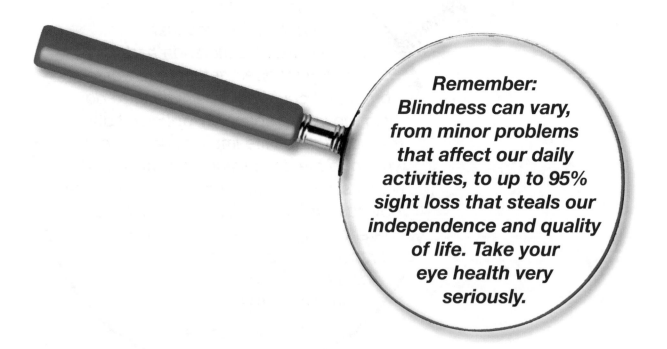

Remember: Blindness can vary, from minor problems that affect our daily activities, to up to 95% sight loss that steals our independence and quality of life. Take your eye health very seriously.

10 Step™ Eye Health Plan - Steps 3 & 4

Proper Nutrition and Diet

Proper Nutrition and Diet can be very confusing to the average person. Earlier, you read the list of vitamins and minerals that should be in our daily diets, but even if they are, you may not be absorbing them properly. You also read that too many starchy and sugary foods will produce too much glucose, which will cause problems in our cells and affect our eyesight.

There are two problems:

1. You have most likely not been fully educated to know the range of ill affects improper nutrition has on your health, as well as the positive effects that may be realized by changing your eating habits to ensure you receive proper nutrition.

2. The other problem is even more of a challenge. Starchy carbohydrates and sugars are addictive, just like any drug. And just like any drug, foods high in sugars and starchy carbohydrates should be avoided. This can be quite difficult, as foods you wouldn't expect to be high in sugar content have a great deal of sugar in them. For example, a can of baked beans has as much as eight teaspoons of sugar. To learn more about the negative impact sugars and starchy carbohydrates have on your health, I recommend going to ReallyHealthFoods.com to discover more.

What it comes down to is this: if you want your life to change, you will need to change your life. As difficult as it may be, I ask that you leave these foods out of your diet for a few months—or at least seriously cut down on them—until you give your eyesight the best possible chance to recover. I have provided the information you need in the Data Sheets in the Appendix, and you can always write to us for further help and information.

Steps 3 and 4 Proper Nutrition and Diet Actions—These may be the most difficult actions to implement, but you can make slow, steady changes for continual progress and recovery.

1. Cut down completely, if possible, or at least significantly on all breads, grains, cereals, biscuits, pastries, potatoes, pasta, corn, sugars, and processed foods for at least the period of your 10 Step™ Plan. Note: sprouted wheat bread is permitted (see Data Sheets).

2. The ideal nutrients for your eyes are contained in vegetables and fruit, nuts, seeds, and beans. All of the proteins, carbohydrates and sugars your body needs are contained in these foods. I also recommend our "Eyesight Soup" as a substitute for breakfast or lunch (see the Appendix for the recipe and ReallyHealthFoods.com).

Page 89.

10 Step™ Eye Health Plan - Step 5

Oxygen and Exercise

Oxygen and exercise go together perfectly to help your eyes for a number of reasons. You read earlier that you need nutrients, such as ATP which helps energize cell regeneration and cleans out your system. Your body also needs oxygen, the most critical element for your health and survival. You need to improve your oxygen uptake to help the regeneration of cells and your eye recovery by exercising and learning to breathe correctly.

Exercise also improves the movement of the fluids in your lymphatic system, helping to get rid of the waste as your cells regenerate. Your whole metabolism will speed up. Your heart will get healthier, and you will feel better (honestly). For your eyes' sake, do it. Get a friend to exercise with you. Relearn diaphragmatic breathing from a singing teacher or yoga class, which is very beneficial for your eyes. You may also want to get the "Breath of Life." (See the Appendix for a supplement to improve your oxygen uptake called OxySorb, especially if you cannot exercise.)

Step 5 Oxygen Actions—Exercise and breathing,either one of which will help you. Together, they can transform your future quality of life at any age. This was proven with 85-year-old residents of a nursing home.

1. Learn your new breathing pattern and practice it often. Every hour (when you're drinking your glass of water) count 100 breaths to get—and stay—in practice. This will help prepare you for aerobic exercise.

2. Exercise for up to 1 hour, 4 times per week. Do exercises that will raise your heart rate to your target heart rate, or 180 beats per minute less your age. For example, if you are 75 years old, your target heart rate is 105 beats per minute (180-75=105). (The "Rebounder" is a very easy home exerciser. See the Appendix for details.)

3. The very least you should do is to take up fast walking and build up to 2 to 3 miles every day. Listen to music, tapes, or ask a friend to go with you to make it fun and enjoyable.

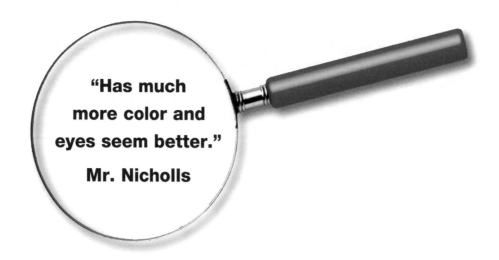

"Has much more color and eyes seem better."

Mr. Nicholls

10 Step™ Eye Health Plan - Step 6

Other Recommended Nutrients

Other recommended nutrients proven to help for all eye diseases are listed below. While they may not be considered critical, it is very difficult not to recommend them, when a person's eyesight is at stake. They include:

a. **Gingko and Bilberry**—These are already contained in the Lutein formula described earlier, but you may buy these separately. The main benefit is support for your veins and arteries, especially when they have been "leaking," and your body needs to rebuild the wall of its veins.

b. **Vitamin A as Beta Carotene and Vitamin C** are particularly good, compatible nutrients. Studies have shown they help the health of the eyes (especially regarding cataracts). Although they are in the "Liquid Vitamins and Minerals formula" listed in the Appendix, people with eye problems will need extra Vitamin C (2-4 grams per day) and Vitamin A (25,OOOIU per day), both of which should be built-up slowly in divided doses.

c. **R-Alpha Lipoic Acid (ALA)**—Studies show particularly good results with ALA in the treatment of glaucoma, diabetic neuropathy, and cataracts. It also helps protect your cells from glycation (glucose poisoning). (Take as directed.)

d. **Dietary Enzyme Supplements** are essential for good digestion as you get older. Studies show that 70-year-olds have only 20% of the enzymes found in a typical 20- year-old. Supplementation, as well as improving the digestion of nutrients, also increases glutathione synthesis and helps protect against free radical ravages. You need to take a good enzyme complex before each cooked meal. Follow the labels when taking them, but make sure the ones you choose are derived from plant—not animal—sources.

e. **Lycopene (another carotenoid,** primarily found in cooked tomatoes or juice) is known to protect eyes against age-related disease. This is also found in the more colorful vegetables that are red, yellow, orange, and green and can be also be taken as a helpful supplement.

10 Step™ Eye Health Plan - Step 7

Detoxify and Cleanse

Detoxifying and cleansing your body is vital to improving the quality of your health. For thousands of years, just about every great physician used herbs (or fasted) to cleanse and support the body's organs.

Step 7 Detoxify and Cleanse Actions include avoiding starchy and dairy foods. By increasing the number of vegetables and fruits you consume, you will start to clean out your body. There are some basics you can easily implement to help your liver as well. We do not recommend fasting, unless under the supervision of an experienced practitioner. Once every year, you should cleanse your system.

1. Take an herbal cleanse that will clean out all the organs of your body over a 2-3 month period (one month for future cleanses). Any detoxifiers/cleanses that promise results in less than 30 days should be avoided. An example of a good herbal formulation can be found in the Appendix.

2. You will need to take another herb for about a month or so to help support and to heal your liver. This well known herb is called Milk Thistle. More details can be found in the Appendix.

3. Last, but not least, you need to restore your digestive system's natural immune system. This inefficiency is why elderly people are sometimes more susceptible to food poisoning. You will need to supplement with "friendly bacteria," which are sometimes called probiotics. These are the healthy bacteria living in your intestines and are responsible for numerous functions, including helping the absorption of taurine, killing food poisoning bacteria, and many others. Details on the friendly bacteria are in the Appendix, along with a sample product recommendation.

10 Step™ Eye Health Plan - Step 8

Homeopathy

Homeopathy has been used for over 100 years to treat eye diseases, as well as many other conditions. It does not conflict with any of the steps here and is relatively easy. We suggest you go to a qualified practitioner and find out specifically what you need. They will ask you several questions about yourself, before suggesting the best solution for you. The good news is that when they find your individual solution, it will work quite quickly, usually within a few weeks.

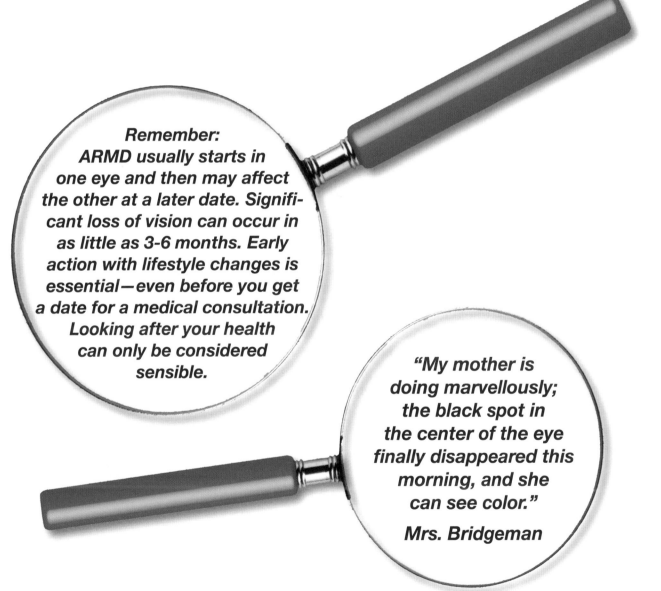

Remember:
ARMD usually starts in one eye and then may affect the other at a later date. Significant loss of vision can occur in as little as 3-6 months. Early action with lifestyle changes is essential—even before you get a date for a medical consultation. Looking after your health can only be considered sensible.

"My mother is doing marvellously; the black spot in the center of the eye finally disappeared this morning, and she can see color."

Mrs. Bridgeman

10 Step™ Eye Health Plan - Step 9

Chelation Therapies

Chelation therapies (oral and intravenous) deal with the treatment and prevention of diseases involving the blood vessels of the body, which directly affects your vision and causes ARMD.

Other diseases related to the blood vessels of the body include coronary artery disease, cardiovascular disease (precursors to stroke), peripheral vascular disease (a diabetes side effect and a precursor to gangrene), eye diseases, and cerebral-vascular disease (precursor to stroke and dementia). These are the major causes of disability and death in the world today.

The traditional approach to these diseases relates to surgery and drugs. However, a case of severe hardening of the arteries need not lead to bypass surgery, heart attack, amputation, stroke, or senility. Oral chelation therapy utilizes a serrapeptase/nattokinase formulation that is gaining popularity due to its ability to clean out the arteries in about three to four months. It is also famous for stopping inflammation of all kinds, particularly in the veins and arteries.

This, combined with the lifestyle changes we indicate in this book, should result in a fast clearing of all blockages to your circulatory system, particularly in the eyes.

The second regime includes the use of ozone and/or a chemical called EDTA (ethylene diamine tetracetic acid) and has been used to help treat diseases mentioned herein.

Intravenous chelation therapy, administered by a properly trained professional and given in conjunction with lifestyle and dietary modification, is an option to be seriously considered by those suffering from coronary artery disease, cerebral vascular disease, brain disorders resulting from circulatory disturbances, generalized atherosclerosis and related ailments that lead to senility and accelerated physical decline.

Clinical benefits from chelation therapy vary with the total number of treatments received and with the severity of the condition being treated. More than 75% of patients treated have shown significant improvement from chelation therapy. More than 90% of patients receiving 35 or more treatments have benefited, when they have also corrected dietary exercise and smoking habits (both of which are known to aggravate arterial disease). Symptoms improve, blood flow increases to diseased organs, the need for medication decreases, and the quality of life improves.

10 Step™ Eye Health Plan - Step 10

MicroCurrent Stimulation or Electronic Acupressure

MicroCurrent stimulation or electronic acupressure are simply different terms for, basically, the same technique which has been used in Europe by the medical profession and natural health practitioners for the past 50 years. The general public in the UK, Europe, and the USA have used them for the past 25 years, often with remarkable results. Electronic Acupressure is being used daily both in Europe and the USA for such diverse treatments as arthritis, sinusitis, asthma, and stroke recovery. It is famous for its good results with eye diseases, thanks to the pioneering work by doctors in the USA, who spotted its potential and got very excited when quite remarkable results were experienced.

In addition to its use for treating eyesight problems, there are 160 different conditions/ailments listed in the book "Simply a Safer Way," which is included with the HealthPoint™.

Step 10 Actions—MicroCurrent Stimulation Actions—It is important, but not necessary, that you consider purchasing a MicroCurrent Stimulator. You can then start treating your eyes, as well as any other conditions from which you may be suffering.

To treat your eyes with this device is quite simple. It is a matter of moving a probe around the edge of the eye socket to find the points that give a tingle. The recommended device is called HealthPoint™. Full details are given in the Appendix, both for ordering the device and instructions for its use. You will find, as have many thousands of others, that once you start using HealthPoint™, it becomes a friend with whom you do not want to part.

Treat the acupuncture points around the eye shown in the data instruction sheets in the Appendix. These can be treated 1-3 times per day. Each point gets treated for approximately 15-30 seconds.

Treat the major acupuncture points shown on the face and the rest of the body. These can be treated, preferably, once a day (or twice a week minimum).

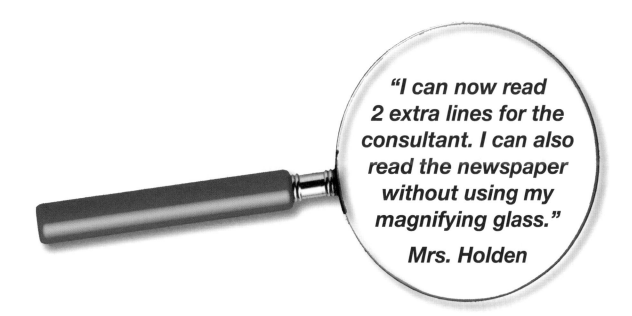

"I can now read 2 extra lines for the consultant. I can also read the newspaper without using my magnifying glass."

Mrs. Holden

"*I knew that her eyes were getting better, but the smile on the face of her optician confirmed it even before the report clearly showed a big improvement.*"

Mrs. Holden

"*I can now see the TV much better, but I still cannot read and I am determined to keep going to be able to read.*"

Mrs. Bolland

"**One of my mother's eyes has improved substantially, although the other is still blind. She feels much better now that there is a solution for her eyes.**"

Mrs. Williams

Appendix Contents

1. Specific Action Plans for conditions listed below:

2. Data Sheets and Resources for Each of the 10 Steps™

Action Plan for Macular Degeneration (Wet or Dry)

Lutein Nutritional Sublingual Spray	+	Microcurrent Stimulation	+	Liquid Taurine	+	EFAs	+	Anti Oxidant Formula	+	MSM Eyedrops

Lutein Nutritional Sublingual Spray is a liposomal spray that contains high levels of the key carotenoids Lutein and Zeaxanthin, together with 22 vitamin and minerals identified in a major study as being essential for eye health. They have been shown to protect the retina against sunlight and oxidative damage by free radicals, strengthen the blood vessels and improve blood flow to the eye. Sprayed under the tongue, it is the most effective way to deliver these nutrients to the eye in a few minutes..

Recommended dosage: 4 sprays 3 times per day for the first 3 bottles then reduce to 2 sprays 3 times per day.

MicroCurrent Stimulation uses a gentle cotton bud probe to safely apply a tiny electrical impulse to the acupressure points around the eyes. Stimulates ATP and cellular regeneration and has been shown in studies to improve the overall success.

Recommended use: Stimulate appropriate MicroCurrent Points shown in the Appendix - 2 treatments per day for the first 2-4 weeks and once per day thereafter.

Liquid Taurine offers better absorption than capsules. Studies have shown Taurine to reduce the oxidative damage caused by sunlight to the eyes. It helps stimulate the body's ability to clean up waste by-products that accumulate in the retina.

Recommended dosage: 8 sprays per day for the first month, and then 2 per day thereafter.

Essential Fatty Acids in liquid form must contain at least 480mg of DHA and 720mg of EPA per teaspoon. This helps improve circulation, integrity of blood vessels, brain function, flexibility, and permeability of cell membranes. It also helps protect the retina's photoreceptor cells.

Recommended dosage: 2 teaspoons per day.

Highly Recommended Antioxidant Formula - Astaxanthin, an extremely powerful antioxidant that is particularly recommended for preventing damage to the retina caused by strong sunlight. Studies show that it is many times more effective than Vitamin E and Beta-Carotene.

Recommended dosage: 3 x 5mg capsules per Day

MSM+Silver Water Drops are recommended for all eye conditions and are an inexpensive self treatment.

Action Plan for Glaucoma

Ocular Lutein Formula Spray	+	Microcurrent Stimulation	+	Alpha Lipoic Acid	+	EFAs	+	Liquid Vitamins & Minerals	+	Anti Oxidant Formula	+	MSM Eyedrops

Ocular-Lutein Formula Spray is a sublingual spray containing Coleus Forskohlii, Lutein, Zeaxanthin, Vitamin B3, and Vitamin E. This is the best product for delivering these specific nutrients to the eye. Studies have shown that these nutrients can help to improve sight and prevent vision loss due to glaucoma. Coleus Forskohlii stops the inflammation that can cause glaucoma. Lutein and Zeaxanthin filter light and serve as potent free radical scavengers for the eye. Vitamin B3 (Niacin) improves blood flow, and Vitamin E is a powerful antioxidant.

Recommended dosage: 6-8 sprays per day for the first two months; then 3 sprays per day for the next two months; and lastly, 1 spray per day as a preventative.

MicroCurrent Stimulation uses a gentle cotton bud probe to safely apply a tiny electrical impulse to the acupressure points around the eyes. Stimulates ATP and cellular regeneration and has been shown in studies to improve the overall success.

Recommended use: Stimulate Appropriate MicroCurrent Points shown in the Appendix - 2 treatments per day for the first 2-4 weeks, and once per day thereafter.

Alpha Lipoic Acid is the only antioxidant that is both fat and water-soluble. Studies have shown that patients with glaucoma have benefited with enhanced color vision and generalized visual sensitivity. It has also been found to reduce diabetic cataract formation and enhance the action of Glutathione and vitamins E and C.

Recommended dosage: 100mg 3 times per day.

Essential Fatty Acids in liquid form must contain at least 480 mg of DHA and 720 mg of EPA per teaspoon. This helps improve circulation, integrity of blood vessels, brain function, flexibility, and permeability of cell membranes. It also helps protect the retina's photoreceptor cells.

Recommended dosage: 2 teaspoons per day.

Essential Liquid Vitamins and Minerals are 3 times more absorbent than tablets, ensuring better utilization by the body, and replaces your current vitamin/mineral formula. This includes the critical minerals selenium and chromium, as well as many others that will help your recovery.

Recommended dosage: ½ oz with breakfast and with your evening meal.

Highly Recommended Antioxidant Formula - Astaxanthin, an extremely powerful antioxidant that is particularly recommended for preventing damage to the retina caused by strong sunlight. Studies show that it is many times more effective than Vitamin E and Beta-Carotene.

Recommended dosage: 3 x 5mg Capsules per Day.

MSM+Silver Water Drops are recommended for all eye conditions and are an inexpensive self treatment.

Action Plan for Cataracts

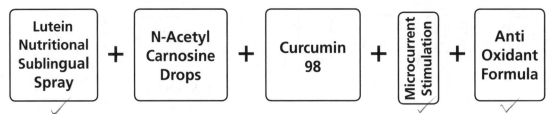

| Lutein Nutritional Sublingual Spray | + | N-Acetyl Carnosine Drops | + | Curcumin 98 | + | MicroCurrent Stimulation | + | Anti Oxidant Formula |

Lutein Nutritional Sublingual Spray is a liposomal spray that contains high levels of the key carotenoids Lutein and Zeaxanthin, together with 22 vitamin and minerals identified in a major study as being essential for eye health. They have been shown to protect the retina against sunlight and oxidative damage by free radicals, strengthen the blood vessels and improve blood flow to the eye. Sprayed under the tongue, it is the most effective way to deliver these nutrients to the eye in a few minutes.

Recommended dosage: 4 sprays 3 times per day for the first 3 bottles then reduce to 2 sprays 3 times per day.

N-Acetyl Carnosine Drops—Stimulates Glutathione directly in the eye and helps dissolve cataracts, and is crucial in stopping free radical damage. Studies have shown that all lenses with cataracts contain approximately 1/5th the amount of Glutathione, as compared to healthy lenses.

Recommended dosage: 6-8 drops per day.

Curcumin98 Capsules—Stimulates Glutathione and offers protection against cataract formation and is crucial in stopping free radical damage. Studies have shown that all lenses with cataracts contain approximately 1/5th the amount of Glutathione, as compared to healthy lenses.

Recommended dosage: 6 caps per day of 95% pure Curcumin.

MicroCurrent Stimulation uses a gentle cotton bud probe to safely apply a tiny electrical impulse to the acupressure points around the eyes. Stimulates ATP and cellular regeneration and has been shown in studies to improve the overall success.

Recommended use: Stimulate appropriate MicroCurrent points shown in the Appendix—2 Treatments per day for the first 2-4 weeks and once per day thereafter.

Vitamin C, Plant Sourced is specifically to help reduce cataracts. Researchers report that a "significant interaction" was observed between age, vitamin C intake, and the prevalence of cataracts.

Recommended dosage: 3 x 1.3 gram capsules per day (1 with each meal).

Action Plan for Diabetic Retinopathy

Liquid Taurine	+	Pancreas Support Spray	+	Lutein Nutritional Sublingual Spray	+	Microcurrent Stimulation	+	EFAs	+	Alpha Lipoic Acid	+	MSM Eyedrops

Liquid Taurine offers better absorption than capsules. Studies have shown Taurine to reduce the oxidative damage caused by sunlight to the eyes. It helps stimulate the body's ability to clean up waste by-products that accumulate in the retina.

Recommended dosage: 8 sprays per day for the first month, and then 2 per day thereafter.

Pancreas Support Spray contains two important trace minerals, Vanadium and Chromium, plus the herb Gymnema Sylvestre, which studies have all shown to be effective with helping diabetes. Note that you should monitor your need for insulin or tablets, as these nutrients may lower or replace the need for these drugs.

Recommended dosage: 6 sprays per day for the first two months; then 3 sprays per day for the next two months; and lastly, 1 spray per day as a preventative.

Lutein Nutritional Sublingual Spray is a liposomal spray that contains high levels of the key carotenoids Lutein and Zeaxanthin, together with 22 vitamin and minerals identified in a major study as being essential for eye health. They have been shown to protect the retina against sunlight and oxidative damage by free radicals, strengthen the blood vessels and improve blood flow to the eye. Sprayed under the tongue, it is the most effective way to deliver these nutrients to the eye in a few minutes.

Recommended dosage: 4 sprays 3 times per day for the first 3 bottles then reduce to 2 sprays 3 times per day.

MicroCurrent Stimulation uses a gentle cotton bud probe to safely apply a tiny electrical impulse to the acupressure points around the eyes. Stimulates ATP and cellular regeneration and has been shown in studies to improve the overall success.

Recommended use: Stimulate appropriate MicroCurrent points shown in the Appendix—2 Treatments per day for the first 2-4 weeks, and once per day thereafter.

Essential Fatty Acids in liquid form must contain at least 480 mg of DHA and 720 mg of EPA per teaspoon. This helps improve circulation, integrity of blood vessels, brain function, flexibility, and permeability of cell membranes. It also helps protect the retina's photoreceptor cells.

Recommended dosage: 1 teaspoon per day.

Alpha Lipoic Acid is the only antioxidant that is both fat and water-soluble. Studies have shown that patients with diabetes have increased cellular uptake and burning of glucose by approximately 50%. It has also been found to enhance the action of Glutathione and vitamins E and C.

Recommended dosage: 100 mg 3 times per day.

MSM+Silver Water Drops are recommended for all eye conditions and are an inexpensive self treatment.

N.B. The above plan, combined with the diet change shown in section 4, can reverse the effects of Type 2 Diabetes (age related).

Action Plan for Floaters

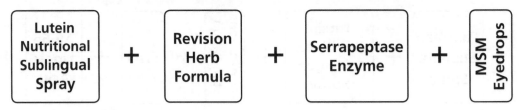

Lutein Nutritional Sublingual Spray is a liposomal spray that contains high levels of the key carotenoids Lutein and Zeaxanthin, together with 22 vitamin and minerals identified in a major study as being essential for eye health. They have been shown to protect the retina against sunlight and oxidative damage by free radicals, strengthen the blood vessels and improve blood flow to the eye. Sprayed under the tongue, it is the most effective way to deliver these nutrients to the eye in a few minutes.

Recommended dosage: 4 sprays 3 times per day for the first 3 bottles then reduce to 2 sprays 3 times per day.

Revision Herb Formula contains Western and Chinese Herbs in a tincture taken orally to help improve blood circulation and eliminate stagnation of "energy" to the eyes. This is done by cleansing and supporting the liver, which according to Chinese medicine, is responsible for the health of the eyes.

Recommended dosage: 1-2 droppers-full 3 times per day for treatment; and 2 times per day for prevention. Do not use as eye drops.

Serrapeptase Enzyme is specifically to help remove non-vital proteins and clear out the eye.

Recommended dosage: 3 per day on an empty stomach (up to 9 may be taken if finances allow).

MSM+Silver Water Drops are recommended for all eye conditions and are an inexpensive self treatment.

Action Plan for Retinitis Pigmentosa

Lutein Nutritional Sublingual Spray	+	Microcurrent Stimulation	+	Liquid Taurine	+	EFAs	+	R-Alpha Lipoic Acid	+	MSM Eyedrops

Lutein Nutritional Sublingual Spray is a liposomal spray that contains high levels of the key carotenoids Lutein and Zeaxanthin, together with 22 vitamin and minerals identified in a major study as being essential for eye health. They have been shown to protect the retina against sunlight and oxidative damage by free radicals, strengthen the blood vessels and improve blood flow to the eye. Sprayed under the tongue, it is the most effective way to deliver these nutrients to the eye in a few minutes.

Recommended dosage: 4 sprays 3 times per day for the first 3 bottles then reduce to 2 sprays 3 times per day.

MicroCurrent Stimulation uses a gentle cotton bud probe to safely apply a tiny electrical impulse to the acupressure points around the eyes. Stimulates ATP and cellular regeneration and has been shown in studies to improve the overall success.

Recommended use: Stimulate appropriate MicroCurrent points shown in the Appendix—2 Treatments per day for the first 2-4 weeks, and once per day thereafter.

Liquid Taurine offers better absorption than capsules. Studies have shown Taurine to reduce the oxidative damage caused by sunlight to the eyes. It helps stimulate the body's ability to clean up waste by-products that accumulate in the retina.

Recommended dosage: 8 sprays per day for the first month, and then 2 per day thereafter.

Essential Fatty Acids in liquid form must contain at least 480 mg of DHA and 720 mg of EPA per teaspoon. This helps improve circulation, integrity of blood vessels, brain function, flexibility, and permeability of cell membranes. It also helps protect the retina's photoreceptor cells.

Recommended dosage: 2 teaspoons per day.

R-Alpha Lipoic Acid is the only antioxidant that is both fat and water-soluble. Studies have shown that it is able to repair oxidative and free radical damage and its protective effect extends to nearly every cell in the body. It has also been found to enhance the action of Glutathione and vitamins E and C.

Recommended dosage: 100 mg 3 times per day.

MSM+Silver Water Drops are recommended for all eye conditions and are an inexpensive self treatment.

Action Plan for Conjunctivitis

Lutein Nutritional Sublingual Spray	+	MSM Eyedrops	+	Colloidal Silver	+	Microcurrent Stimulation	+	EFAs

Lutein Nutritional Sublingual Spray is a liposomal spray that contains high levels of the key carotenoids Lutein and Zeaxanthin, together with 22 vitamin and minerals identified in a major study as being essential for eye health. They have been shown to protect the retina against sunlight and oxidative damage by free radicals, strengthen the blood vessels and improve blood flow to the eye. Sprayed under the tongue, it is the most effective way to deliver these nutrients to the eye in a few minutes.

Recommended dosage: 4 sprays 3 times per day for the first 3 bottles then reduce to 2 sprays 3 times per day.

MSM+Silver Water Drops are recommended for all eye conditions and are an inexpensive self treatment.

Colloidal Silver - Conjunctivitis may be caused by infection; use Hydrosol silver as eye drops to help heal the problem (use Hydrosol Silver as eye drops and alternate hourly with MSM+Silver Water Drops).

MicroCurrent Stimulation uses a gentle cotton bud probe to safely apply a tiny electrical impulse to the acupressure points around the eyes. Stimulates ATP and cellular regeneration and has been shown in studies to improve the overall success.

Recommended use: Stimulate appropriate MicroCurrent points shown in the Appendix—2 Treatments per day for the first 2-4 weeks, and once per day thereafter.

Essential Fatty Acids in liquid form must contain at least 480 mg of DHA and 720 mg of EPA per teaspoon. This helps improve circulation, integrity of blood vessels, brain function, flexibility, and permeability of cell membranes. It also helps protect the retina's photoreceptor cells.

Recommended dosage: 2 teaspoons per day.

Action Plan for Multiple Sclerosis Eye Problems

Lutein Nutritional Sublingual Spray	+	Microcurrent Stimulation	+	Serrapeptase Enzyme	+	EFAs	+	Curcumin 98	+	MSM Eyedrops

Lutein Nutritional Sublingual Spray is a liposomal spray that contains high levels of the key carotenoids Lutein and Zeaxanthin, together with 22 vitamin and minerals identified in a major study as being essential for eye health. They have been shown to protect the retina against sunlight and oxidative damage by free radicals, strengthen the blood vessels and improve blood flow to the eye. Sprayed under the tongue, it is the most effective way to deliver these nutrients to the eye in a few minutes.

Recommended dosage: 4 sprays 3 times per day for the first 3 bottles then reduce to 2 sprays 3 times per day.

MicroCurrent Stimulation uses a gentle cotton bud probe to safely apply a tiny electrical impulse to the acupressure points around the eyes. Stimulates ATP and cellular regeneration and has been shown in studies to improve the overall success.

Recommended use: Stimulate appropriate MicroCurrent points shown in the Appendix—2 Treatments per day for the first 2-4 weeks, and once per day thereafter.

Serrapeptase Enzymes is specifically to help non-vital proteins and help clear out the eye.

Recommended dosage: 3 per day on an empty stomach.

Essential Fatty Acids in liquid form must contain at least 480 mg of DHA and 720 mg of EPA per teaspoon. This helps improve circulation, integrity of blood vessels, brain function, flexibility, and permeability of cell membranes. It also helps protect the retina's photoreceptor cells.

Recommended dosage: 2 teaspoons per day.

Curcumin 98 is a high strength extract of the spice Turmeric, which promotes the production of glutathione, the body's major antioxidant. It is recommended for the prevention of cataracts and uveitis and has been widely used in the treatment of M.S.

Recommended dosage: 6 per day (2 before each meal) for the first month; then 3 per day thereafter.

MSM+Silver Water Drops are recommended for all eye conditions and are an inexpensive self treatment.

Action Plan for Computer Fatigue Syndrome

Lutein Nutritional Sublingual Spray	+	VIVA-Eye	+	Pinhole Massager Glasses	+	MSM Eyedrops	+	Microcurrent Stimulation

Lutein Nutritional Sublingual Spray is a liposomal spray that contains high levels of the key carotenoids Lutein and Zeaxanthin, together with 22 vitamin and minerals identified in a major study as being essential for eye health. They have been shown to protect the retina against sunlight and oxidative damage by free radicals, strengthen the blood vessels and improve blood flow to the eye. Sprayed under the tongue, it is the most effective way to deliver these nutrients to the eye in a few minutes.

Recommended dosage: 4 sprays 3 times per day for the first 3 bottles then reduce to 2 sprays 3 times per day.

VIVA-Eye adds vitamin A directly to the eye. This acts as a lubricant, preventing irritation and dryness caused by insufficient blinking, dry air (air conditioning), and possible free radicals radiated from the computer screen.

Recommended dosage: 1-3 drops per day as needed.

Massager Pin Hole Glasses can improve blood flow and relieve eyestrain and headaches caused by computer work, farsightedness, nearsightedness and Presbyopia. Pinhole Massager Glasses can relax tired eyes, build up the flexibility of your eyes, and can, in some cases, reduce your current prescription.

Recommended use: 5-10 minutes twice per day.

MSM+Silver Water Drops are recommended for all eye conditions and are an inexpensive self treatment.

MicroCurrent Stimulation uses a gentle cotton bud probe to safely apply a tiny electrical impulse to the acupressure points around the eyes. Stimulates ATP and cellular regeneration and has been shown in studies to improve the overall success.

Recommended use: Stimulate appropriate MicroCurrent points shown in the Appendix—2 Treatments per day for the first 2-4 weeks, and once per day thereafter.

Action Plan for Dry Eyes/BLEPHARITIS

Lutein Nutritional Sublingual Spray	+	VIVA-Eye	+	Microcurrent Stimulation	+	EFAs	+	Vision Tone Herbs	+	Thera Tears	+	MSM Eyedrops

Lutein Nutritional Sublingual Spray is a liposomal spray that contains high levels of the key carotenoids Lutein and Zeaxanthin, together with 22 vitamin and minerals identified in a major study as being essential for eye health. They have been shown to protect the retina against sunlight and oxidative damage by free radicals, strengthen the blood vessels and improve blood flow to the eye. Sprayed under the tongue, it is the most effective way to deliver these nutrients to the eye in a few minutes.

Recommended dosage: 4 sprays 3 times per day for the first 3 bottles then reduce to 2 sprays 3 times per day.

VIVA-Eye adds vitamin 'A' directly to the eye. This acts as a lubricant, preventing irritation and dryness caused by insufficient blinking, dry air (air conditioning) and possible free radicals radiated from the computer screen.

Recommended dosage: 1-3 drops per day as needed.

MicroCurrent Stimulation uses a gentle cotton bud probe to safely apply a tiny electrical impulse to the acupressure points around the eyes. Stimulates ATP and cellular regeneration and has been shown in studies to improve the overall success.

Recommended use: Stimulate appropriate MicroCurrent points shown in the Appendix—2 Treatments per day for the first 2-4 weeks, and once per day thereafter.

Essential Fatty Acids in liquid form must contain at least 480 mg of DHA and 720 mg of EPA per teaspoon. This helps improve circulation, integrity of blood vessels, brain function, flexibility, and permeability of cell membranes. It also helps protect the retina's photoreceptor cells.

Recommended dosage: 2 teaspoons per day.

Essential Vision Tone Herb Formula includes a combination of Western and Chinese herbs to strengthen the eyes.

Recommended dosage: ½ dropper full 2 times per day on an empty stomach. Do not take as eye drops.

Severe conditions need TheraTears which have been shown to restore conjunctival goblet cells and corneal glycogen levels in dry eyes. This is very effective for post-LASIK surgery patients suffering from dry eyes.

Recommended dosage: 1-3 drops per day as needed.

MSM+Silver Water Drops are recommended for all eye conditions and are an inexpensive self treatment.

Action Plan for General Vision Problems

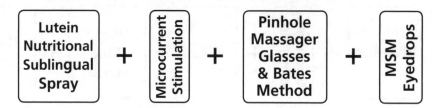

Lutein Nutritional Sublingual Spray is a liposomal spray that contains high levels of the key carotenoids Lutein and Zeaxanthin, together with 22 vitamin and minerals identified in a major study as being essential for eye health. They have been shown to protect the retina against sunlight and oxidative damage by free radicals, strengthen the blood vessels and improve blood flow to the eye. Sprayed under the tongue, it is the most effective way to deliver these nutrients to the eye in a few minutes.

Recommended dosage: 4 sprays 3 times per day for the first 3 bottles then reduce to 2 sprays 3 times per day.

MicroCurrent Stimulation uses a gentle cotton bud probe to safely apply a tiny electrical impulse to the acupressure points around the eyes. Stimulates ATP and cellular regeneration and has been shown in studies to improve the overall success.

Recommended use: Stimulate appropriate MicroCurrent points shown in the Appendix—2 Treatments per day for the first 2-4 weeks, and once per day thereafter.

Massager Pin Hole Glasses can improve blood flow and relieve eyestrain and headaches caused by computer work, farsightedness, nearsightedness and Presbyopia. They can relax tired eyes, buildup the flexibility of your eyes and can, in some cases, reduce your current prescription.

Recommended use: 5-10 minutes twice per day.

Bates Method - is a method of exercising and improving sight developed by William Bates. It can be found in many books in the health stores and book shops and is now on DVD (e-mail us at info@eyesight.nu).

MSM+Silver Water Drops are recommended for all eye conditions and are an inexpensive self treatment.

1. RECOMMENDED NUTRITION DATA SHEETS

Lutein Sublingual Spray - Essential Eye Nutrition

MACULAR DEGENERATION is the number one cause of blindness in our aging population. Worldwide, many millions of people currently suffer from this retinal disorder that obscures central vision. Approximately 25% of people over age 65 have some manifestation of Age-Related Macu-lar Degeneration (ARMD).

Lutein and Zeaxanthin were identified in 1995 as the only two carotenoid antioxidants specific to lens and macula health. Selectively accumulated from plasma and deposited in the lens, macula, and lungs, Lutein and Zeaxanthin filter light and serve as potent free radical scavengers for the retina. The macular pigment, composed of Lutein and Zeaxanthin, functions as a color filter to protect the light-sensitive photoreceptor cells, which are responsible for visual acuity, from UV-light originated free radical damage.

Studies in 1997:

- Showed a 30% reduced macular pigment density in eyes with ARMD.

- Found a correlation between reduced macular pigment density and increased lens density (cataracts) in seniors.

- Demonstrated that macular pigment density can be increased with dietary and/or supplementing with Lutein.

Maintaining sufficient levels of Lutein and Zeaxanthin, the only carotenoid antioxidants active in the retina, can prevent ARMD, cataracts, and preserve youthful visual sensitivity.

The natural health industry is committed to bringing you the most effective nutritional supplement formulations, based upon the most recent scientific research, and the highest quality of product ingredients available. To that end, there is now a Lutein/Zeaxanthin formulation, which is in a sublingual form. (We discussed earlier why that is so important to absorption.) That formulation was developed in 1996. In 2006 the formula was further enhanced by the addition of a range of key vitamins and minerals to make it one of the most powerful eyesight formulas available. The objective was to formulate a dietary supplement based on the most recent "peer review" research, to impede the progress of macular degeneration.

The Lutein formulation spray was designed to meet the specific need of the senior population, and a liposomal sublingual delivery system was chosen to eliminate the problem of poor gastrointestinal absorption in the elderly. The results have far exceeded the expectations of all those concerned.

The results have far exceeded the expectations of all those concerned.

Over the past four years, doctors and their patients in the USA have used adjectives like "miraculous" to describe improvements, after using the Lutein formulation spray for a brief 2-6 months. Visual improvements reported include reduced glare and visual fatigue, better contrast, color, night vision, adaptability, and a sharper view.

"Most individuals supplementing with sublingual Lutein and Zeaxanthin report reduced glare and visual fatigue, better contrast, color perception, night vision, adaptability, and a sharper view."

The Latest Lutein Study

Results of the the latest exciting Lutein study presented at ARVO 2002 meeting by:
S.P. Richer (1), W.Stiles (1), L.Statkute (2), K. Y. Pei (1), J.Frankowski (1), J.Nyland (1), J.Pulido (3), D.Rudy (4). (1 - Eye Clinic, DVA Medical Center, North Chicago, IL; 2 - Cook County Hospital, Chicago, IL; 3 - Eye and Ear Infirmary, UIC, Chicago, IL; 4 - Family Medicine, FUHS/Chicago Medical School, North Chicago, IL, USA.).

Main Findings:

❖ Average eye Macular Pigment Optical Density (MPOD) increased 50% in both the Lutein and Lutein plus antioxidant treatment groups

❖ Significant improvement in multiple measures of visual function, including distance/near acuity and contrast sensitivity (CSF) in both treatment groups, with the Lutein plus antioxidant group displaying a broader improvement in CSF.

❖ Crossover, double crossover, and video-documentation pre- and post-treatment were consistent with improvement in outcome measures.

Conclusions:

Reversibility of AMD symptoms has important biophysical, physiological, and clinical implications.

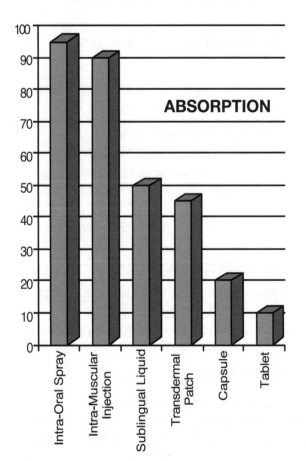

This clinical trial agrees with previous studies suggesting ARMD to be a nutrition-responsive disorder. The authors believe that low technology visual evaluation protocols, combined with Lutein-based nutritional intervention recommendations, may improve the eye health of older patients with the dry form of ARMD.

2 fluid oz. Intra-Oral Sublingual Spray; 30-Day Therapeutic Supply, 53-Day Maintenance Supply.

Active absorption at therapeutic dose:

Lutein	10mg
Zeaxanthin	2.5mg
Taurine	5mg

together with 21 natural nutrients recommended for eye health

Other Ingredients:
Purified Water, Glycerine, Natural Flavors, Lecithin, Vitamin E

Dosage:

12 sprays per day, reducing to 6 after 3 bottles.

Best taken a minimum of 10 minutes after liquids and 1 hour after food. Spray Lutein under the tongue and hold for 2 minutes. Allow 10 minutes before food or drink.

Why is Lutein Absorption a Concern (especially as we get older)?

The human eye requires more nutrition and oxygen to maintain healthy tissue and function than any other organ in the body! Presently, we are witnessing new breakthroughs in helping to prevent vision loss. The National Institute of Health (NIH) in the USA is studying 4,600 people to follow the effects of nutritional supplementation in relation to cataracts, macular degeneration, and glaucoma. The study is identifying "which" supplements are most important and "how" these nutrients should be taken.

Oftentimes, we know the therapeutic dosage for a specific condition, but we do not know how much of the prescribed nutrient is absorbed into the bloodstream via the gastrointestinal system when taken orally by tablet, capsule, or gel cap. We do know that after the age of 40, and continuing on as we age, our gastrointestinal absorption rate reduces significantly, according to studies. This problem becomes even more serious, when combined with health conditions or digestive disorders that further reduce absorption, such as ulcers, diverticulitis, acid reflux, dysbiosis, etc.

Again, it's not how much you take, but how much your body tissues absorb that is important. With a higher level of absorption, more nutrients reach their intended destination, thereby requiring a lower dosage intake. More nutrients in a pill or capsule are not necessarily better. What is important is how we can best ensure the uptake of recommended "therapeutic dosages."

One way around this problem is to take nutritional supplements using the most efficient delivery system available. The most important nutrients should be taken in the form of sprays when available. Spraying inside the mouth (intra-oral) or under the tongue (sublingual) has the best absorption rate.

The following table compares absorption rates of delivery systems. It is taken from the PDR (The Physicians Desk Referenc):

Delivery System	Rate of Absorption	Delivery System	Rate of Absorption
Pill or tablet	10%	Sublingual Liquid	50%
Capsule	20%	Intra-muscular Injection	90%
Gel Cap	30%	Intra-oral or Sublingual Spray	95%
Trans-dermal Patch	45%	Intravenous Injection	100%

Intra-oral and sublingual sprays have become a viable solution with the introduction of liposomes. Liposomes hold both water and fat-soluble nutrients in little fat containers to provide an efficient transport system that allows for maximum absorption by the body. These fat containers bypass the stomach and take a quicker more efficient route by slipping through the mucosal membrane under the tongue and directly into the bloodstream, as shown in studies. The intra-oral or sublingual spray method of delivery is also very helpful for individuals who have difficulty swallowing pills or capsules and, since a lower dosage of nutrients is required, it is cost effective.

There are a good many products on the market that contain Lutein and various other ingredients that are beneficial for the eyes. Many contain 'the AREDS' formula. This is a list of vitamins and minerals that were identified by the Age Related Eye Disease Study as being important nutrients. So how can you decide which one to take? We have seen that when sprayed under the tongue, nutrients absorb 9 times better than tablets, so look at the ingredient list on the packet and divide by 9 before comparing the quantity with a sublingual spray. Then you can compare the cost per mg of the key ingredients Lutein and Zeaxanthin (If it does not have any, do not waste your money). Remember that you require 10 mg of Lutein per day to help your eyes recover.

I have compared most of those on the market and have never found one that is better value for money and effectiveness than MaxiFocus™.

References:

❖ Weiner, Dietz & Laue, Senile changes in absorption and elimination processes and their importance in pharmacotherapy, Zeitschrift fur Alternforschung/Journal of ageing Research, (ZFA), 38(5):355-60, Sep-Oct 1983.

❖ Dietz, Lane & Laue, Digestion and absorption in the elderly, ZFA, 33(1): 65-78, 1978. Scarpace, J. Am. Geriatr Soc, Decreased receptor activation with age, 36(11):1067-71, 1988 Nov.

❖ Baker, Jaslow & Frank, Severe impairment of dietary folate utilization in the elderly, J Am Geriatr Soc, 26(5):218-21, 1978 May. Physicians' Desk Reference, NPPDR No. 18:676, 1997.

❖ Liposomes a practical approach. RRC New Editor, IRL press at oxford university press. 1990. Liposome technology, Gregodadis Ed. Vol 1, 11, 111. 2nd Edition, CRC Press, 1993.

❖ Elias Fattal, Technological aspects of liposomes preparation, University of Paris-Sud, School of Pharmacy, URA CNRS 1218, Chatenay-Malabry, France. Weiner, Dietze & Laue, Age-dependent alterations of intestinal absorption. Arch Gerontol Geriatr, 3(2):97-108, 1984 Jul.

❖ Scientific American, 256 (1):103-111, 1987.

Essential Fatty Acids—FOCUS ON DHA & EPA

Both Omega-3 and Omega-6 fatty acids are essential nutrients for normal development in mammals. Omega-6 fatty acids are necessary primarily for growth, reproduction, and the maintenance of skin integrity. Omega-3 fatty acids are involved in the development and function of the retina and cerebral cortex and other organs, such as the testes. (1)

Docosahexanoic acid (DHA) and eicosapentaenoic acid (EPA) are essential Omega-3 fatty acids found in abundance in cold water fish and their oils. DHA is an essential nutrient for achieving optimal brain and eye function. (2) It comprises about 60% of the rod outer segments in the photoreceptor cells with which we see. (3) Brain tissue is about 60% fat, 25% of which is DHA. DHA levels correlate with visual and mental performance and several neurological and visual disorders, including retinitis pigmentosa.

Cells in the retina, brain, and other parts of the nervous system have connecting arms that transport electrical currents, sending visual information from the retina to the brain and messages from the brain throughout the body. DHA supplementation ensures the optimal composition of cell membranes necessary for the most effective transmission of these signals. Plentiful stores are needed, and a daily dose of approximately 500 mg daily is recommended, if taken by capsule.

A 1990 study demonstrated that DHA with EPA given in the form of fish oil exerts a beneficial dose-dependent effect on coronary circulation with reduced triglycerides, total cholesterol, and blood pressure, while causing no significant increase in bleeding time. (4) Its use in wet macular degeneration is unparalleled, since its main work in the body is to heal and support blood vessel walls.

Evening primrose, borage, and blackcurrant oil are good sources of Omega-6 essential fatty acids, including gamma-linolenic acid (GLA). Supplementation with GLA may offer a method to bypass the disturbance in Omega-6 essential fatty acid metabolism associated with diabetes and diabetic retinopathy. (5)

DHA and EPA are found in abundance in fish oil supplements, many of which are in stores.

If you prefer a vegetarian solution, then consider what is being called "The Master of Oils"— Hemp Seed Oil. As well as being beneficial taken by mouth, it will even have a health effect just massaged into the skin and being absorbed into the body (and healing most skin problems— eczema, psoriasis, etc.).

Note: Fatty acids are an essential part of every person's diet, whatever their age.

1. Connor WE; Neuringer M.; Prog Clin Biol Res; 1988: 282; 275-94.

2. Neuringer M, Anderson 3. J., Connor WE, "The essentiality of n-3 fatty acids for the development and function of the retina and brain," Ann Rev Nutr., 1988; 8: pp/l 7-41.

3. Salem et. al., 1996; P Martinez et al, 1992).

4. Haglund et. al., "Effects of a new fish oil concentrate on triglycerides, cholesterol, fibrinogen and blood pressure" Nutritional Research 1990; 227:347-53.

5. Jamal GA, "The Use of Gamma Linolenic Acid in the Prevention and Treatment of Diabetic Neuropathy," Diabetic Med 111994; 11:145-49.

Nutrients
(Colloidal Minerals, Major Minerals & Vitamins)
Minerals & Vitamins per ounce

Supplement	Amount per Serving	Daily Value %
Calcium (Tricalcium Phosphate Citrate)	600mg	50
Choline Bitartrate	25mg	*
Chromium (Chromium Polynicotinate)	200mcg	167
Copper (Copper Gluconate)	2mg	100
Folic Acid (Vit B Conjugate)	500mcg	125
Inositol	50mg	*
Magnesium (Citrate Gluconate Concentrace)	300mg	50
Manganese (Manganese Gluconate)	10mg	500
Organic Seleniumethionine	200mcg	286
Potassium (Potassium Gluconate)	250mg	12.5
Vit A (Palmitate)	5000IU	100
Vit A (Beta Carotene)	5000IU	100
Vit B1 (Thiamin Mononitrate)	3mg	200
Vit B12 (Methylcobalamin)	6mcg	100
Vit B2 (Riboflavin)	3.4mg	200
Vit B3 (Niacinamide)	40mg	200
Vit B5 (Calcium Pantothenate)	20mg	200
Vit B6 (Pyridoxine Hydrochloride)	4mg	200
Vitamin C (Ascorbic Acid)	300mg	500
Vit D (Cholecalciferol)	400IU	100
Vit E (Alpha Tocopheryl Acetate)	60IU	200
Vit K (Phytonadione)	80mcg	100
Zinc (Zinc Oxide)	15mg	100
Trace minerals	600mg	*
Phosphorus (Amino Acid Chelate)	190mg	19
Iodine (Potassium Iodide)	150mcg	100
Biotin	300mcg	100
Boron (Sodium Borate)	2mg	*
Molybdenum (sodium)	75mcg	100
Chloride Concentrate	102mg	3
Amino Acid Complex	10mg	*
Aloe Vera (200:1)	2mg	*

Organic Colloidal Minerals

Each fl oz contains1250mg of the following 70+ natural colloidal minerals

Antimony	Neodymium
Arsenic	Nickel
Aluminium Hyd	Niobium
Barium	Nitrogen
Beryllium	Osmium
Bismuth	Oxygen
Boron	Palladium
Bromine	Phosphorous
Cadmium	Platinum
Calcium	Potassium
Carbon	Praseodymium
Cerium	Rhenium
Cesium	Rhodium
Chloride	Rubidium
Chromium	Ruthenium
Cobalt	Samarium
Copper	Scandium
Dysprosium	Selenium
Erbium	Silicon
Europium	Silver
Fluorine	Sodium
Gadolinium	Strontium
Gallium	Sulphur
Geranium	Tantalum
Gold	Tellurium
Hafnium	Terbium
Holmium	Thallium
Hydrogen	Thorium
Indium	Tin
Iodine	Titanium
Iron	Tungsten
Lanthanum	Ytterbium
Lead	Yttrium
Lithium	Zinc
Lutetium	Zirconium
Magnesium	
Manganese	
Molybdenum	

Take 1-3 fl oz just before breakfast and/or evening meal

Taurine Spray

Active Ingredients (per bottle):

❖ **Taurine**

Taurine is a sulphur-containing amino acid found naturally in egg whites, meat, fish, and milk. High concentrations are found in the heart muscle, white blood cells, skeletal muscle, and central nervous system.

In the retina, there are two binding proteins specific to Taurine; intracellular concentrations are higher in the retina than in any other region derived from the central nervous system.

Taurine plays a role in the process of rhodopsin, regeneration necessary for night vision. It is essential to the retinal pigment epithelium and the photorecep-tors (cells that we see with), where it is found at levels ten times higher than other free amino acids. Taurine helps protect cell membranes from oxidative attack. It helps transport nutrients across cell membranes, acts as a catalyst to retinal cells that remove cellular debris, and assists in the elimination of potentially toxic substances. Taurine, in combination with retinol, protects lipids twice as much as retinol alone. Taurine protects rod outer segment lipids during exposure to cyclic light.

Diabetes increases the retina's requirements for Taurine. Glucose rapidly and specifically decreases Taurine content in retinal pigment epithelial cells. Uptake of Taurine is increased in the retina and retinal pigment epithelium with higher levels of Insulin and glucose concentrations. Taurine also appears to protect the lens against the development of "sugar cataracts" by an antioxidant effect.

A deficiency state of Taurine is often associated with an imbalance in intestinal flora. This condition, dysbiosis, is commonly called "leaky gut" and inhibits Taurine absorption. Lowered levels of Taurine may also be associated with cardiac arrhythmias, disorders of platelet formation, an overgrowth of Candida, physical or emotional stress, a zinc deficiency, and excessive consumption of alcohol.

It is also important to note that the drugs chlorpromazine, a tranquillizer, and chloroquine, an antimalarial/antiinflammatory agent, inhibit the uptake of Taurine and have been known to cause retinal damage with prolonged or excessive dosage.

Daily supplementation of Taurine Spray is advised, at least until the digestive tract health is restored (Probiotics, Cleanse, Digestive Enzymes etc.) taken by capsule. Taurine Spray is available in a 2 oz. spray bottle (320 sprays) and will be absorbed even before the digestive tract probiotics are restored

Astaxanthin

Astaxanthin is possibly the most potent natural antioxidant ever discovered. AstaXanthin (asta-zan-thin) has tremendous promise for health and well-being. Research suggests that it is up to 500 times more powerful than vitamin E and 10 times more powerful than beta-carotene.

What is it? AstaXanthin is a carotenoid pigment that occurs naturally in marine microalgae. It is also what makes salmon and prawns pink.

What does it do? AstaXanthin:

❖ Crosses the blood brain barrier and is 1 of only 4 antioxidants known to do so.

❖ Inhibits the destruction of the fatty acids and proteins in the cell membrane and the mitochondrial membranes in the cells caused by peroxidation of fats.

❖ Traps more types of radicals (alkoxyl, hydroxyl, peroxyl, and singlet and triplet oxygen).

❖ Because it binds to a lipid (fat) protein, it travels more readily in the body and is more available for use.

❖ Inhibits reactive oxygen species that causes inflammation to the cells, thus producing anti-inflammatory capabilities.

❖ Provides superior protection against UVA light-induced oxidative stress.

❖ Enhances the actions of vitamins C and E in the body.

What are the Benefits?

❖ Protects the eye from sunlight

❖ Scavenges the free radicals from other sources that cause damage to the eyes and other organs.

❖ Beneficial against diabetes by preserving the beta cells in the pancreas

❖ Can inhibit Helicobacter pylori infection in the digestive tract

❖ May inhibit the growth of some tumors

Superior Antioxidant Properties of R-Alpha Lipoic Acid

R-Alpha Lipoic Acid (ALA), a vitamin-like substance found in foods and produced by the body in limited amounts, may be the most valuable of all the antioxidant nutrients. In addition to neutralizing both oxygen and nitrogen free radicals, ALA has been studied for its ability to actually repair oxidative damage, to regenerate other antioxidants and chelate excess metals.

ALA is one of many substances produced by the body in large quantities in young people, but production declines with age. Health-conscious individuals may inadvertently limit their intake of this important nutrient by reducing their intake of red meat, one of the richest dietary sources of ALA. Lipoic acid deficiency has been linked to muscle wasting, brain atrophy, and increased lactic acid accumulation. Lower serum levels of Lipoic acid are frequently found in patients with cirrhosis of the liver, diabetes, and heart disease.

ALA Works in Both the Watery and Fatty Areas of the Cells

Unlike other antioxidants, ALA is both hydrophilic (water soluble) and lipophylic (fat soluble), enabling it to act both inside the cell and in the intracellular spaces. Because of its universal solubility, ALA is able to neutralize both hydroxyl and singlet-oxygen free radicals, two of the most dangerous types, wherever they are found. It works to prevent free radical damage regardless of whether it is in the brain fluids, blood, stored fat, the heart, pancreas, kidneys, liver, bone or cartilage. Its protective effects extend to virtually every cell in every organ and tissue.

These characteristics enable ALA to easily cross the blood-brain barrier and increase brain energy. It has been shown to improve long-term memory in aged mice, probably by preventing free radical damage to cell membranes. Other studies support a neuro-protective role against various chemicals.

ALA—DHLA: Two Antioxidants in One

ALA supplements actually give you two antioxidants in one. As ALA does its work, it is reduced to Dihydrolipoic Acid (DHLA), another important antioxidant that can deactivate peroxyl and other types of free radicals. When DHLA is oxidized, it reverts back to ALA. The molecule goes back and forth automatically in the body, accomplishing many important and beneficial functions.

DHLA Regenerates Other Antioxidants

In order to deactivate free radicals, antioxidants must give up an electron. Therefore, their effective "life" is limited. DHLA is able to restore the missing electrons and extend the life of other antioxidants. It replenishes vitamin C and indirectly recycles vitamin E, so those antioxidants remain active longer. Supplemental ALA also helps maintain a normal ratio of reduced to oxidized Co-enzyme Q10. In addition, ALA and DHLA provoke the cell to produce significantly higher levels of glutathione, the indispensable cellular antioxidant synthesized within the mitochondrion.

Protective Effect of ALA on the Liver

Burt Berkson, M.D., Ph.D., author of "The Alpha Lipoic Acid Breakthrough," believes ALA to be an excellent therapeutic agent for many types of liver disorders. In his book, he describes how administering intravenous ALA saved the lives of four people who suffered severe liver damage after eating poisonous mushrooms. Two weeks later, the patients' liver function tests were normal and they felt fine. In-vitro studies indicate that ALA may be beneficial to patients with acute and chronic alcohol toxicity.

ALA is also an effective chelating agent for mercury, arsenic, copper, excess iron, cadmium, excess calcium, zinc, and lead. Excesses of these metals can overwhelm the liver's detoxification system, increase free radicals and oxidative stress, and cause serious damage to tissues and organs.

A Co-Enzyme in Sugar Metabolism

ALA also functions as a co-enzyme in sugar metabolism. In a study of adult diabetic patients, ALA increased cellular uptake and burning of glucose by approximately 50%. In two double blind, placebo-controlled trials, ALA significantly reduced symptoms of diabetic peripheral neuropathy (pain, burning, paresthesia, and numbness) in the feet and improved cardiac autonomic dysfunction in insulin dependent diabetics. In both lean and obese diabetic patients, ALA also prevents hyperglycemia-induced increments of serum lactate pyruvate levels, and it increases insulin sensitivity and glucose effectiveness.

Muscle Strength and Energy

ALA speeds the body's breakdown and burning of sugar, which occurs primarily in muscle cells. Efficient burning of glucose is essential for normal muscle energy. A 33-year-old woman who suffered a genetic defect affecting cellular energy production was treated with ALA. Glucose uptake, glucose burning, muscle-energy metabolism, and muscle strength increased, as documented by laboratory tests. Since ALA can increase energy levels in muscle cells, it may be valuable in sports nutrition and weight control.

Cardiovascular Health

Because of its antioxidant capabilities and its ability to boost glutathione production and recycle other antioxidants, ALA can also play a role in cardiovascular health. Both ALA and DHLA are extremely powerful for deactivating peroxynitrite, a particularly dangerous type of free radical formed by a combination of superoxide radicals and nitric oxide. It contributes to the development of Atherosclerosis, lung disease, neurological disorders, and chronic inflammation, such as that associated with rheumatoid arthritis and inflammatory bowel disease. Ischemic reperfusion injury results from the large number of free radicals generated when blood flow is restored after surgery. ALA treatment before and after reperfusion can lessen or prevent such injury to the heart, brain, and peripheral nerve tissues.

Immune Function Support

In a pilot study, supplementation with 150 mg of Lipoic acid 3 times a day was shown to increase plasma ascorbate, glutathione and T-helper cells, and to optimize the ratio of T-helper cells to T-suppressor cells. Other studies have demonstrated that Lipoic acid also helps to inhibit HIV replication by decreasing the activity of reverse transcriptase. Apoptosis (programmed cell death) is triggered by cellular oxidation and can be prevented.

Cataracts

Based on animal experiments, ALA may have value in preventing cataracts that are caused by oxidative stress in the lens. Since ALA is both water soluble and fat-soluble, it can get deep into the eye tissues and destroy free radicals that cause protein changes resulting in cataracts. Animals given chemicals to induce cataracts had a 60% reduction in cataract formation when treated with ALA.

Radiation and Chemotherapy

Russian scientists who treated children exposed to radiation after the nuclear incident in Chernobyl reported ALA, used by itself or with vitamin E, to be an effective treatment for radiation poisoning. They noted that abnormal liver and kidney functions were also corrected. ALA has been shown to protect the bone marrow of mice from radiation injury, has been reported to neutralize the toxic effects of radiation in animals and to alleviate the harmful effects of cancer chemotherapy in humans.

Pancreas Support

Any Synergistic Formulation needs Gymnema Sylvestre, the only substance scientifically shown to regenerate Pancreatic B-cells

GYMNEMA SYLVESTRE

Recent statistics reveal that the average American is consuming 145 lbs. of sugar a year—more if you include sugar from carbohydrates, etc. The results of this sugar binge are: hyperinsulinemia, hyperlipidemia, obesity, cardiovascular disease, diabetes, Syndrome X, A.G.E. products, cataracts and various forms of neuropathy. These are the chronic diseases of our times. The frontline organ dealing with this glucose onslaught is the pancreas. The increasing levels of diabetes and dysglycemia problems are indicators that the pancreas is not up to dealing with this level of sweetness.

Gymnema sylvestre, a woody climber from the tropical forests of India, has been shown to repair, revitalize and regenerate the pancreas. In one study, Streptozotocin was used to induce diabetes in rats. Gymnema treated rats had increased insulin secretion and beta cell numbers. There was no effect on normal rats. Rabbits induced with diabetes using Alloxan showed the same results. In tests in humans with both Type I and Type II diabetes, Gymnema was shown to be effective. Gymnema extract was able to reduce blood glucose, glycated haemoglobin, glycosylated plasma proteins whilst increasing C-peptide levels and conventional diabetic drug therapy. These effects are not noted with conventional therapy. All patients developed secondary hypoGlycaemic symptoms and had to have their drug dosages reduced after several weeks.

When tested on healthy Individuals, Gymnema does not produce any acute reduction in fasting blood glucose levels. This research is starting to overturn the conventional concept that the pancreatic beta cell damage in juvenile, maturity-onset and experimentally-induced diabetes is irreversible.

Gymnema extract has the ability to normalize blood glucose function by repairing, revitalizing and regenerating the beta cells of the pancreas. Gymnema in traditional Indian medicine is known as a stomachic, diuretic, and diabetic controller. In Sanskrit it's known as Meshashringi and in Hindi, Gurmar. Both names refer to its ability to destroy sugar. Gymnema has the interesting properly of being able to stop sweet taste. This property was investigated in the early 1900s a crude fraction known as "gymnemic acid." This fraction not only stopped sweet taste but also glycouria. Modern research has isolated a polypeptide, gurmarin that is responsible for stopping the sweet taste. Several triterpenpoid saponins have been isolated that have the blood glucose regulating effect.

VANADYL SULPHATE

Vanadyl sulphate, a salt of the mineral vanadium (vanadium oxysulphate), has demonstrated insulin-like effects on glucose metabolism in both animal and human trials. Clinical trials have shown a significant decrease in Insulin requirements by patients with insulin-dependent diabetes mellitus after Vanadyl sulphate therapy and a significant decrease in cholesterol levels in both insulin-dependent and non-insulin-dependent diabetics. There was an increase in basal mitogen-activated protein and S6 kinase activities in mononuclear cells from both groups that mimicked the effect of insulin stimulation in controls. Vanadyl sulphate given to diabetic rats stimulates glucose uptake and metabolism leading to glucose normalisation. Rats with Streptozotocin-induced diabetes were given Vanadyl sulphate for three weeks. Although insulin levels were still depressed, glucose tolerance was normalized.

Vanadyl Sulphate has also been shown to lower high blood pressure in the same rats, as a result of the reduction in excess insulin. Vanadyl Sulphate is likely to be beneficial for diabetes mellitus. It partially restored insulin production in diabetic rats' pancreas tissue. Three weeks of Vanadyl Sulphate treatment, followed by 13 weeks without it, still protected the size and insulin content of pancreas islets. It also maintained glucose tolerance regardless of insulin levels. In another study on diabetic rats, Vanadyl Sulphate maintained the normal levels of glucose, lipids, creatinine, and thyroid hormone. It also corrected abnormalities in heart function and in glycerol output from adipose tissue.

Muscle cells show increased intake of glucose, amino acids and insulin. Muscles increase tissue formation and retention. Less protein from muscles is available for fuel, so the body turns to fat for fuel. As the metabolic rate increases, the muscles' sensitivity to Vanadyl appears to increase. Glycogen production is increased in muscle and liver cells. The result—less fat, more muscle, and more endurance.

NIACIN (B-3)

Vitamin B3, also called Niacin, Niocinamide, or Nicotinic Acid, is an essential nutrient required by all humans for the proper metabolism of carbohydrates, fats, and proteins, as well as for the production of hydrochloric acid for digestion. B3 also supports proper blood circulation, healthy skin, and aids in the functioning of the central nervous system. Because of its role in supporting the higher functions of the brain and cognition, vitamin B3 also plays an important role in the treatment of schizophrenia and other mental illnesses. Lastly, adequate levels of B3 are vital for the proper synthesis of insulin, and the sex hormones, such as estrogen, testosterone, and progesterone.

Chromium taken with niacin has been found to be a synergistic combination that increases glucose utilization beyond that when taking Niacin or Chromium alone.

CHROMIUM POLYNICOTINATE

Research in recent years has been published showing that chromium in its nontoxic, trivalent state bound in an organic complex with nicotinic acid as Glucose Tolerance Factor (GTF) improves insulin function. Most chromium used as a GTF supplement comes from Brewer's yeast. Chromium in Brewer's yeast is in the Polynicotinate form. Chromium Polynicotinate is up to 300% more bio-available than chromium picolinate.

Chromium doesn't stimulate the increase of insulin, but rather acts in potentiating the action of the hormone. Human trials have shown that Chromium works in the following ways: reduces fasting glycemia, mean blood glucose and glycated hemoglobin. It lowers cholesterol and triglycerides but less than the other indices.

Newer research points to chromium as being able to sensitize tissues to Insulin. This action would be beneficial in insulin resistance and Syndrome X problems. Chromium not only acts in glucose related problems, but is also involved in body composition and fat distribution. In double-blind studies, just the addition of chromium supplementation, with no other dietary changes, altered the body fat composition to increase nonfat body mass.

One factor affecting chromium stores in the body is the amount of sugar that an individual consumes. Once chromium has acted as a cofactor in insulin response, it is excreted in the urine. With the high sugar diet of today, the turnover rate of chromium is quite high. Patients with the highest risk for developing diabetes need chromium the most. The highest tissue stores of chromium occur in newborns. As the result of diet and sugar stress, chromium is depleted from the body as we age. Studies have shown that diabetics have lower plasma chromium levels than non-diabetics.

Niacin-bound chromium is more bio-available than chromium picolinate. A recent animal study at the University of California found that Chromium Polynicotinate was absorbed and retained up to 311% better than chromium picolinate and 672% better than chromium chloride

Gymnema Sylvestre	890mg
Niacin (B-3)	288mg
Methylsulfonylmethane (MSM)	96mg
Boron Chelate	80mg
Chromium Polynicotinate	384mcg
Vanadyl Sulphate	224mcg

Pancreas Support Spray
1 fluid oz. Bottle Intra-Oral Sublingual Spray
30 to 53 day Supply

Remember:
The eye has a greater requirement for nutrients and oxygen compared to any organ in the body, and even a slight lack of these essential nutrients and/or blood flow can cause an immediate deterioration (as shown in times of tension head-aches and stress) in eye function.

"I can now see the TV, even with my bad eye. Everything is brighter and clearer."

Mrs. Rawes

EYE EASE HERBAL FORMULATION
helps ease conjunctivitis and sties

Recommended dosage is ½ dropper-full 3 times a day taken BY MOUTH for treatment when infection is present. Best taken on an empty stomach.

Note: These drops are not eye drops, and should be taken internally only, unless used with a compress. If used as a compress, here are the preparation instructions:

Make 8 ounces of boiling water. Put in 1 dropper-full of EyeEase. Let the alcohol burn off for one minute then let the water cool down till its warm. Proceed to dip in a washcloth and place over your closed eyes.

Burdock root (Arctium lappa) is a liver tonic and lymphatic cleanser. Herbalists have traditionally used burdock for skin conditions, such as sties, boils and carbuncles.

Forsythia (Forsythia suspensa), recognized in Traditional Chinese Medicine as a "cooling" herb, has been shown to inhibit viral and bacterial infections, including staphylococcus, streptococcus and salmonella.

Goldenseal (Hydrastis canadensis) is gaining popularity for its natural, yet potent, antibiotic and antiseptic qualities. Herbalists have prescribed it for more than hundreds of years to treat inflammation of the eyes.

Echinacea (Echinacea Angustifolia) is one of the most popular immune boosters. It not only supports the body's ability to fight its own battles by enhancing our immune response, but it also has its own antibacterial and antiseptic qualities.

Honeysuckle (Lonicerae japonicae), like forsythia, clears the "heat" of infection and inflammation and alleviates the swelling of sties. A natural antibiotic, it has been shown to inhibit viral and bacterial infections, including staphylococcus, streptococcus and salmonella.

Chrysanthemum Flower (Chrysanthemum marifoli) is used in the treatment of many eye conditions for its antibiotic effect. It is useful in relieving heat in the eyes, such as in the conditions of sties and conjunctivitis.

Eyebright (Euphrasia officinalis) has been shown since the Middle Ages as a universal eye remedy for both internal and external inflammatory conditions.

Chamomile (Matricaria chamomilla) is a very effective herb, when used externally as a compress to help with inflammatory conditions of the eye.

Red Raspberry Leaf (Rubus idaeus) is an astringent herb that helps to break up excess mucous in the eyes.

Marigold, also referred to as Calendula (Calendula officinalis), is a very effective herb in the treatment of inflammatory conditions when used externally (taken internally it aids digestion).

Related Diseases to be helped: Blepharitis, Conjunctivitis, Sties

TheraTears

TheraTears from Advanced Vision Research. Shown to restore conjunctival goblet cells and corneal glycogen levels in the dry eyes. This is very effective for post-LASIK surgery patients suffering from dry eyes. No preservatives.

Recommended use is to start with 4 vials per day, and then as needed. Each individual's need varies, so you must determine optimum usage for yourself.

Dry Eyes

Myth: Dry eyes are just a condition of eyes.

Fact: The eyes often reflect a larger problem that needs to be treated systemically.

Overview:

Dry eyes, often referred to as Dry Eye Syndrome, is the most frequent patient complaint to eye doctors. Many millions in all groups experience varying degrees of dry eye syndromes. Like most eye conditions, Dry Eye Syndrome is often related to health conditions in the rest of the body. It is commonly associated with dryness of other mucous membranes, interior body surfaces, such as joints and brittle nails. It can also be a sign of digestive imbalances or of more serious systemic autoimmune diseases, such as rheumatoid arthritis, Sjogrens syndrome or lupus erythematosus.

The proper production of tears basically takes place at three layers:

1. The Mucus Layer—is the closest layer to the corneal epithelium. It is produced by the conjunctival goblet cells, and is absorbed by the corneal surface glycoproteins, creating a hydrophilic corneal surface.

2. The Aqueous Layer—is between the Mucous and Lipid Layers, and comprises 90% of the tear film's thickness. It is secreted by the lacrimal gland and incorporates all water-soluble components of the tear film (slightly alkaline at pH of 7.4).

3. The Lipid Layer—is the most superficial layer. It is produced by the Meibomiam glands with minor contribution from glands of Zeis and Moll. The secretion is a sebaceous material that is fluid at body temperature, and retards evaporation of the aqueous layer and lowers surface tension, thereby allowing tear-film to mold itself to the eye's surface.

Blinking renews the tear film by delivering aqueous and lipid to tear film and sweeping away debris. The normal blink interval is every 5 seconds. Tear film is typically stable for about 10 seconds.

Symptoms:

The typical symptoms include dryness, grittiness, irritation, difficulty reading for long periods of time, burning and even the seeming contradiction of excessive tearing or watering.

Causes:

❖ Any disruption in the tear production process as described in the Overview.

❖ Blepharitis can often cause dry eye symptoms due to inflammation of the eyelid margins, which is caused by a bacterial infection (Staphylococci). This condition can compromise the quality of the tear film, causing tears to evaporate more quickly. The bacteria produce waste material that can cause a mild toxic reaction leading to chronic red irritated eyes.

❖ Computer users tend to blink much less frequently (about 7 times per minute vs. a normal rate of around 22 times/minute). This leads to increased evaporation along with the fatigue and eyestrain associated with staring at a computer monitor. Ideally, computer users should take short breaks about every 20 minutes to reduce this factor. Also, adjusting the monitor so that it is below eye level will allow the upper lid to be positioned lower and cover more of the eye's surface, again to reduce evaporation.

❖ LASIK surgery temporarily disrupts the ocular surface/lacrimal gland unit. Also, during LASIK, roughly 60-70% of the superficial nerve fibres in the cornea are severed, which impacts sensation and affects aqueous tears. With compromised sensation, the blink rate can slow to the point where the tear film breaks up before the next blink can reconstitute. This may result in mild to severe dry eye syndrome for many months after surgery. This condition usually clears up eventually.

❖ Diseases that may be associated with dry eyes include Rheumatoid Arthritis, Diabetes (especially when the blood sugar is up), Asthma, Thyroid disease (lower lid does not move when blinking), Lupus, and possibly Glaucoma.

❖ Age—tear volume decreases by as much as 60% at age 65 relative to the rate at age 18. Dry Eye Syndrome affects 75% of people over age 65.

❖ Hormonal changes in women can cause decreased tear production brought on by pregnancy, lactation, menstruation, and post-menopause.

❖ Other causes include too much coffee drinking, smoking, wearing contact lenses, air-conditioning or heat.

Drugs that can cause dry eye symptoms:

❖ Antibiotics
❖ Blood Pressure medications
❖ Antidepressants
❖ Over-the-counter Vasoconstrictors (e.g. Visine)
❖ Antihistamines

❖ Birth Control pills
❖ Appetite Suppressants
❖ Ulcer medications
❖ Diuretics

Conventional Treatment:

❖ Artificial Tears: Some form of over-the-counter artificial tears is usually recommended. Although they may provide temporary relief, they merely palliate the symptoms. Worse, the preservatives can aggravate the condition, and can even kill corneal cells. Tears that promise to "get the red out" will reduce circulation in the eye, decrease production of the tear film, and worse, eventually make your eyes even drier.

❖ Punctal Occlusion: Punctal occlusion is a procedure used to help dry eye patients by closing the tear drainage canals with silicone plugs, which keep most of the fluid from the surface of the eye. This may provide long-term relief.

Vision Tone Herbal Formula

Vision Tone Formula—this classic Chinese formula contains; Rehmannia, Cornus, Dioscorea, Alisma, Poria, Moutan, White Peony, Lycium Berry, Chrysanthemum Flower, American Ginseng, Bilberry, Gingko, Licorice, Shou Wu, Wild Yam and Hoelen. It is a historical tonic for visual problems such as cataracts, dry eyes, and light sensitivity.

Recommended dosage is 1/2 dropper-full twice a day for prevention, or 3 times a day for treatment.

Best times to take the herbs are when you get up in the morning, and in the afternoon between 4 P.M. and 6 RM.

Herbs should preferably not be taken with meals.

Note: This formula is only to be taken by mouth. It is not an eye drop.

Other herbs include the following:

American Ginseng (Panax quinquefolium) is a tonic particularly good for the adrenal glands. American ginseng is gentler that the Asian varieties: it has more of a yin function. American ginseng supports the immune system, provides energy, and balances blood sugar levels.

Bilberry (Vaccinium myrtillus) appears to play a significant role in the prevention of cataracts. In one study, a combination of bilberry and vitamin E stopped cataract formation in 97 percent of the patients—without side effects. Bilberry may also strengthen the collagen that supports eye structure. An antioxidant, it protects the lens from oxidation.

Gingko (Ginkgo Biloba) has been shown to increase visual acuity in people with macular degeneration. Ginkgo increases blood circulation to the head, which includes the brain and the eyes, so it can speed healing of all of the tissues associated with vision.

Shou Wu nourishes the system that makes birth, development and maturation graceful. It is a tonifying herb used in this context for fading vision.

Related Diseases to be helped:
Dark Circles Under the Eyes, Dry Eyes and Light Sensitivity

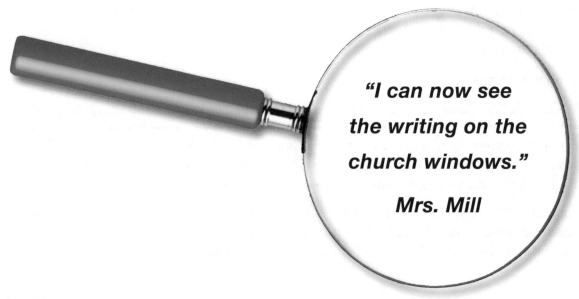

"I can now see the writing on the church windows."

Mrs. Mill

VIVA-DROPS®

Product Features

VIVA-DROPS® is the only ophthalmic lubricant that combines all the following unique characteristics:

❖ Patented formulation. A combination of ingredients, including antioxidants, in a safe and effective formulation.

❖ NO preservatives. Preservatives in eye drops are known to cause irritation and damage normal healthy tear constituents. The formulation and manufacturing process of VIVA-DROPS® achieves microbiological acceptance standards for ocular products, without the need for a preservative.

❖ NO mercuric compounds or anticholinergics. Mercury and anticholinergics in eye drops may cause localized and systemic adverse effects. Some over-the-counter (OTC) lubricant eye drops contain thimerosal. Some homeopathic eye drops contain mercury (mercurius sublimatus) and atropine (belladonna).

❖ Non-oily solution. Formulated for optimum comfort and efficacy.

Ingredients and Product Information

Name: VIVA-DROPS® Lubricant Eye Drops

Product Class: Ophthalmic Lubricant (OTC)

Active Ingredient: Polysorbate 80 (Demulcent and Antioxidant)

Inactive Ingredients: Purified Water (Dilutant)
Sodium Chloride (Tonicity Agent)
Sodium Citrate (Buffering Agent and Antioxidant)
Citric Acid (Buffering Agent and Antioxidant)
EDTA (Chelating Agent and Antioxidant)
Mannitol (Antioxidant)
Retinyl Palmitate (Antioxidant)
Sodium Pyruvate (Antioxidant)

FDA Approved Uses: For use as a lubricant to prevent further irritation or to relieve dryness of the eye.

Directions: Instill 1 or 2 drops in the affected eye(s) as needed.

"Dry eyes" is a very common eye problem, especially in women and elderly patients. It is the primary reason for a patient's inability to wear contact lenses comfortably. Medication and environmental factors are major causes of dry eyes and irritation. Look at the ingredients in VIVA-DROPS® and use with confidence.

ReVision Herbal Formula

ReVision Formula is a classic Chinese herbal formula known to improve blood circulation and "eliminate stagnation of energy" to the eyes.

Related Diseases to be helped:

Blepharospasm, Floaters, Glaucoma, Macular Degeneration, Pterygium, Vitreous Detachment

Dosage:

- Preventative: ½ dropper-full 2 times daily

- Therapeutic: ½ dropper-full 3 times daily

- Best times to take the herbs are when you get up in the morning, and when you go to sleep at night. Best taken on an empty stomach.

Ingredients:

- Herbs include: Atractylodes, Bilberry, Bupleurem, Coleus, Dandelion, Dong Quai, Eyebright, Gardenia, Ginger, Gingko, Hoelen, Licorice, Milk Thistle, Poria, Tree Peony and White Peony.

- Bilberry (Vaccinium myrtillus), the European version of the blueberry, has been called the vision herb for its powerful effect on all types of visual disorders. Research has shown that bilberry can improve night vision, relieve visual fatigue, and help protect the eyes from glaucoma, cataracts, and macular degeneration. Bilberry strengthens the capillaries that deliver oxygen and nutrients to the eyes; feeds eye muscles and nerves, and works as an antioxidant to inhibit damage by free radicals.

- Bupleurem (umbelliferae) "improves the free flow of energy" in the body.

- Coleus (Coleus forskohlii), a member of the mint family, is traditionally used in Ayurvedic medicine. Studies have shown coleus to lower intraocular pressure by relaxing smooth muscles in the eye. Its antihistamine properties may reduce the allergic component of increased eye pressure.

- Dandelion Root (Taraxacum officinalis radix) is a liver tonic, which aids in digestion and the balancing of blood sugar levels necessary for capillary health. In addition, dandelion contains antioxidants to help tissues stay healthy.

- Eyebright (Euphrasis officinalis) has been known throughout history as an effective herb to help tonify the eyes.

- Gardenia (rubiaceae) "reduces heat" in the body, allowing "better free flow of energy."

- Ginkgo Biloba increases circulation to the retina, and has been shown in studies to increase visual acuity in persons with macular degeneration.

- Milk Thistle (Silybum marianum) s an excellent liver tonic. It increases the flow the liver, helping to detoxify poisons in our bloodstream. It nourishes the liver and increases energy throughout the body.

ReVision Formula Sublingual Drops 2 fl. oz. Bottle

Note: This formula is only to be taken by mouth. It is not an eye drop.

Glutathione Stimulation

Essential Glutathione offers protection in cataract formation, and is crucial in stopping free radical damage. Studies have shown that all lenses with cataracts contain approximately one fifth the amount of Glutathione, as compared to healthy lenses.

Glutathione is also one of the body's most important antioxidants. It protects cells from free radical damage, particularly free radicals that are produced naturally by the body's own detoxification process. It can also neutralize free radicals produced by stress, exercise, and cigarette smoking. The body produces glutathione using the trace mineral Selenium plus Cystine, Glycine and Glutamate.

There are 3 easy ways to improve glutathione production (presuming you are already taking a multi-supplement, including selenium, and eating lots of vegetables and fruits):

1. N-Acetyl Cysteine—This is an Amino acid and can be taken in high doses to stimulate Glutathione. It is available in capsule form and needs 2-3 grams per day for best effect. This can cause digestive discomfort but can easily be lowered to an acceptable level for comfort.

2. Curcumin—Is the active ingredient extract in Turmeric (the yellow spice). Turmeric has about 4% Curcumin content, but it is now available as 95% pure Curcumin. This has many benefits, and not just for eyes. Studies are being published for a wide range of conditions, including Alzheimer's, cancer, Crohn's disease, colitis and lung problems.

3. N-Acetyl Carnosine Drops (NAC)—Stimulates Glutathione directly in the eye and helps dissolve cataracts and is crucial in stopping free radical damage. Studies have shown that lenses with cataracts can be cleared in approx. 3 months, according to Russian studies.

See Data Sheets for Curcumin98™ and NAC drops.

Curcumin Treating eye disorders. Curcumin is, apparently, more than your typical kitchen spice. It's the substance that gives ginger its yellowish color, and it has been implicated in the treatment of certain eye diseases and conditions. One of those is known as chronic anterior uveitis (CAU), an inflammatory condition of the vascular layer of the eye, particularly the area comprising the iris. In one small study, Curcumin was given orally to 32 chronic anterior uveitis patients who were divided into two groups. The first group received Curcumin alone, whereas the second group received a combination of Curcumin and antitubercular treatment. Amazingly, all of the patients treated with Curcumin alone improved, compared to a response rate of 86% among those receiving the combination therapy. The researchers concluded that **Curcumin was just as effective as corticosteroid therapy**, the only available standard treatment for chronic anterior uveitis at present, adding that "the lack of side effects with Curcumin is its greatest advantage compared with corticosteroids."

Similar research using rats and rabbits found that Curcumin effectively inhibited chemically induced cataract formation, even at very low dietary levels. The same study also found, for the first time, that this type of induced cataract may be accompanied by apoptosis of epithelial cells in the eye and that Curcumin may lessen the apoptotic effect. In one of the earliest studies examining Curcumin as a potential cataract therapy, researchers fed two groups of rats, diets that included corn oil, or a combination of Curcumin and corn oil, for 14 days. Afterward, their lenses were removed and examined for the presence of lipid peroxidation. The scientists discovered that "the lenses from Curcumin-treated rats were much more resistant to... induced opacification than were lenses from control animals."

Awasthi S, et. a/. Curcumin protects against 4-hydroxy-2-trans-nonenal-induced cataract formation in rat lenses. Am J Clin Nutr 1996 Nov;64(5):761-6. Lai B et al. Efficacy of curcumin in the management of chronic anterior uveitis. PhytotherRes 1999Jun;13(4):318-22. Pandya U etal. Dietary curcumin prevents ocular toxicity of naphthalene in rats. Toxicol Lett 2000 Jun 5;115(3): 195-204.

Remember:
Doing nothing is not an option for those who value their independence and who want to maintain their quality of life. If your doctor disagrees with the current scientific research, and does not support your efforts, then you will need to seek the help of EyeSight Action or a more sympathetic professional.

Remember:
Not all eye doctors know (or agree) that nutrition deficiency is the cause of eye problems. If you believe them and do nothing, then you have no chance for recovery. If you give it a fair 12-month trial, you have a good chance for recovery.

Massager Pinhole Glasses

These glasses are used for two areas of eye health:

1. To improve blood flow to the eyes where additional flow would resolve the effects of tension from computer or tiring driving.

2. Improving blood flow into the eyes and using the pin holes effect to improve eyesight from eye diseases and other vision problems.

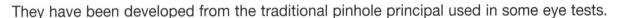

These can help with most focusing problems, even if you already use spectacles or lenses.

They have been developed from the traditional pinhole principal used in some eye tests.

Scientific research has enabled the manufacturers to maximize their vision improvement effect.

Pinhole Massager Glasses consist of conventional spectacle frames with the lenses replaced by opaque screens containing lots of small holes. Looking through the pinholes immediately makes blurred vision sharper. This can help people learn to focus where they had previously needed glasses.

How do Massager Pinhole Glasses Work?

When the eye receives a blurred image, it moves the focus, looking for a sharper image. If this is not found, the eye is left unfocused. With the Pinhole Massager Glasses, the image is slightly clearer so the eye can learn to focus again and exercise the focusing muscles. With regular practice, the eyes are able to see better without glasses.

Use Massager Pinhole glasses (with Lutein Spray and MSM drops) for a few minutes a day to help:

- Low Vision diseases
- Nearsightedness
- Farsightedness
- Presbyopia
- Eye Strain/Headaches
- Computer Stress

Computer Users - Why are computer screens a problem?

The eyes of computer users spend a lot of time focused (staring) at the short distance of the screen. This can be stressful for the muscles, as a result of restricted blood flow around the eyes that can cause a build up of tension around the eyes, leading to sore eyes and even headaches. If it is possible to use Pinhole Massager Glasses while working at the computer they will help the eyes focus more easily allowing them to relax more.

The prolonged close focusing involved with computer use can produce short sight in time.

Watching TV with Massager Pinhole glasses to relax the eyes can avert this tendency.

"Not only did they help eyestrain but they seemed to protect my eyes when I was using the computer. Before they would get bloodshot and itchy after I'd been looking at the screen for a while, but when I used the pinholes, those symptoms no longer occurred." - Maggie

2. MICROCURRENT STIMULATOR DATA SHEETS
Microcurrent Stimulation / Electronic Acupuncture

For helping Age-Related Macular Degeneration and other Eye Diseases

MicroCurrent stimulation (or electro-acupuncture) has been used for the past fifteen years to treat Macular Degeneration and other eye diseases. The initial results obtained by individual doctors in the USA indicate that 70% of patients with the dry or wet form of macular degeneration will have a significant improvement of vision.

There are many factors related to the condition known as Macular Degeneration. The most common cause is the circulation problems that increase as we age. In order to function properly, the macula has a very high requirement for proper nutritional elements, oxygen, and the elimination of waste products. Circulation problems reduce the supply of oxygen and nutrients to the macula and will cause a dysfunction in the macula and ultimately cause degeneration. Electronic stimulation is a therapy in which a weak electric current is used, through points known as acupuncture points, to stimulate the retina and the diseased macula to restore sight.

Dr. Merill Allen and Dr. Leland Michael published their preliminary study in 1993, on the rate of development of ARMD in people using nutritional supplements and simultaneous therapy with electronic stimulation. Dr. John Jarding reported his results in 1997, after treating 35 macular degeneration patients with a controlled electronic stimulation applied to eight points around the eye—all 35 patients reported an improvement in their vision.

An Exciting New Development

An electronic device, researched over 12 years by a leading British doctor, is designed to provide all the benefits of MicroCurrent Stimulation, as well as Electronic Acupuncture (without needles). MicroCurrent stimulation is used by health professionals in many hospitals and is designed to be used safely and effectively by the public for self-treatment.

THIS DEVICE WORKS IN TWO WAYS:

1. With the help of its unique searching system, it enables you to quickly become expert at precisely locating therapy points.

2. The device then applies electrical pulses to these points, enabling you to treat any condition that acupuncture can help.

It is safe, drug-free, has no side effects, and is easy to use.

You will know you are on the correct point when you FEEL a distinct sensation. Mild electric pulses then stimulate these points.

THE EFFECTS OF THIS THERAPY ARE:

❖ An immediate and long lasting relief from at least 60% of the symptoms.

❖ With continuing therapy, promotion of healing and tissue regeneration.

The recommended device is HealthPoint™. (Call the help line, shown at the front of the book, for more information.)

History of Micro Current Stimulation

By Larry Ratliff, President & CEO Dove Alliance USA, Inc.

Back in the late 1960s Dr. Julian Kenyon, a UK surgeon and Master Acupuncturist, had a vision of putting the healing power of acupuncture into the hands of the lay person—and as a consequence, improving the effectiveness of acupuncture.

After twelve years of research, the result was the EPS. As the first micro current device of its kind, the EPS incorporated a locating system that allowed the user to locate acupuncture points with 100% accuracy and then stimulate that point with a very minute electronic pulse. When coupled with traditional acupuncture protocols, the results were remarkable and repeatable.

Dr. Kenyon's research was founded on the works of Robert Becker and others that had been researching the electrical properties of the human body. In the course of his study, Dr. Kenyon recognized an amazing connection between this western research and eastern medicine.

Western research had identified specific channels of electromagnetic energy that correspond exactly to the eastern description of meridians. Also small points exist, in exactly the same location as described acupuncture points, which are 10-40 times more conductive than the surrounding skin. When stimulated electrically, these points demonstrate a direct correlation to the electromagnetic fields in the meridians. The voltages in the meridians can be readily measured and change in relation to health or lack of health. Although the western researchers were not aware of it, they had confirmed the theory of eastern medicine.

Now Dr. Kenyon had a tool to work with and a method of cause and effect evaluation. From this beginning, Dr. Kenyon went on to refine and define the most effective electrical properties and procedures to use when treating the body. It was found that bipolar micro currents, in a range of less than 50 micro-amps, having a square waveform and frequency of 10 hertz, would trigger the body's natural healing system and promote tissue regeneration.

The current generation of the EPS is called HealthPoint™ (or HealthTouch) and has been successfully used in clinics and by lay people around the world for over 20 years.

During the same period of time, it had been discovered that stimulating the body with currents in the milli-amp range could provide relief from some types of pain. As a result, western research was moving forward on devices having much higher output currents. Based on the "gate theory" of pain control, an electrical current is applied to the nervous system and interferes with the transfer of information from one nerve cell to another, preventing a signal from reaching the brain. The pain is there, the condition is there, but the body does not acknowledge it. These high current devices are termed TENS devices and are widely used today for the treatment of many painful conditions.

Continued research has brought information leading to improvements in the hardware and techniques of TENS treatment. This refinement has broadened the field of use of TENS stimulation and, interestingly, reduced the usable output currents down into the micro current range. One of these researchers is Dr. Joel Rossen, an acupuncturist and veterinarian, who had a desire to improve the treatment of animals and had started building his own TENS devices.

As always, necessity is the mother of invention. By 1976 all of the ingredients for a breakthrough in Macular Degeneration treatment were in place, but existed separately and apparently unrelated in an arena that was spurned by leading researchers:

1. Dr. Kenyon had joined micro-current stimulation with acupuncture.

2. TENS research had brought outputs down into the area of micro-currents.

3. Advances in nutrition research were bringing the focus from corrective medicine to preventive lifestyle and good health practices.

Then, in 1979, Grace Halloran entered the picture. Having a great desire to cure her eye problems, an unlikely chain of events transpired to bring about a miracle cure.

Grace had hereditary Retinitis Pigmentosa (RP) and, at the time, was working for a football team as a consultant, specializing in alternative treatment of injuries. Her friend, a physiotherapist, introduced her to Dr. Joel Rossen, who was conducting training classes on the use of his TENS devices. Grace worked with Dr. Rossen for several years refining the unit design. Then a successful treatment for a serious injury to her son prompted her to try the micro-current device on her own eye condition—with some success. Grace continued to refine the treatment procedure, founded the Integrated Visual Healing program, and has been spreading the word ever since.

In 1985, while presenting seminars, Grace came into contact with Dr. Leland Michael and Dr. John Jarding, who conducted a 25-patient study. Then, in 1992-1999 came doctors Wallace, Miller, Khouri, Chee, Kondrot, and Nagel. The word is spreading. Grace is still conducting seminars.

Studies. Early studies were simply clinical trials where the treatment was administered and results recorded. This started with Grace Halloran and continues today with every doctor that provides this treatment protocol. All reports are very consistent in results and safety.

In 1993, Dr. Michael published a paper covering treatment of 25 ARMD patients over a seven-year period. (Dr. Michael died shortly after publication and his practice was taken over by Dr. John Jarding). Dr. Jarding then conducted an investigative trial over a period of seven years, concluding in 2000.

In 1998, Dr. Miller published a statistical analysis of ARMD patients treated with the micro-current protocol.

Dr. Rossen and the Macular Degeneration Foundation are currently conducting an FDA study.

The Doctors. 1976—Dr. Julian Kenyon, 1979—Grace Halloran, 1979—Dr. Joel Rossen, 1985—Dr. Leland Michael, 1985—Dr. John Jarding, 1992—Dr. Jerry Wallace, 1997—Dr. Harry Miller, 1998—Dr. George Khouri, 1998—Dr. Percival Chee, 1998—Dr. Edward Kondrot, 1999—Dr. James Nagel

With the knowledge we now have—there is hope!

Using a combination of nutrition and micro current stimulation, a 60% to 80% improvement in visual acuity on 80% of the patients treated and stoppage of progression has been consistently achieved, with no adverse side effects.

Vision loss can be reversed in the majority of cases, and the progression of the eye disease stopped in the rest. Research goes on, and progress is being made. Reports continue to come in about amazing successes and discoveries.

Treatment Overview

Cotton Bud Instructions

The cotton bud probe provides a comfortable means of stimulating the points around the eye shown on the following pages. For all other body points use the remote gold probe.

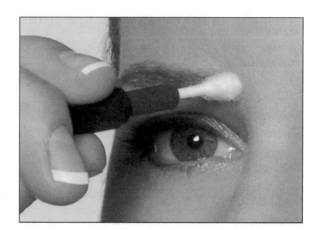

1. Twist Cotton Bud plug into the extension socket on HealthPoint™, ensuring that the cotton is in contact with the metal inner.

2. The person being treated holds the stainless steel plate on the HealthPoint™.

3. Switch HealthPoint™ On.

4. Set Timer switch to Manual.

5. Dip Cotton Bud in a small dish of saline (salt water or small saline dropper bottle from the chemists) made with sea salt.

6. Touch the wet cotton bud to the stainless steel plate and you should get a high-pitched sound if a good contact is made.

7. If good contact, set timer switch to Constant.

8. Treat general points around the eye as per instructions for 30 seconds on each point.

9. Treat other points shown on specific points page for 30 seconds.

10. Each eye point should create a retinal flashing (or away from eyes a small tingle). If the sensation is too strong around the eyes, slide the Intensity switch down to suit.

11. Treat once per day minimum and twice preferably.

12. You cannot overtreat.

13. When renewing the cotton bud, cut the tip off close to the start of the cotton.

Call the help line, shown at the front of the book, for support.

BASIC EYE POINTS TO STIMULATE FOR ALL EYE CONDITIONS

Treatment Points

Treat the ring of 10 points shown in Fig. 1. There are 7 just on the edge of the eye socket and three around the eyebrow (see description below). Use the Cotton Bud Probe as shown in fig. 3 on page 69.

POINT 1 Is on the bony edge of the eye socket, central with the centre of the eye.

POINT 2 Is on the bony edge of the eye approximately halfway to the outer eye corner from Point 1.

POINT 3 Is on the bony edge of the eye approx. 1/2" from the outer edge of the eye.

POINT 4 Is on the bony edge of the socket directly above Point 2

POINT 5 Is on the bony edge of the eye socket directly above Point 1

POINT 6 Is on the bony edge of the eye approx. 1/2" from the inner corner of the eye and Point 5.

POINT 7 Is on the bony edge of the eye socket directly below point 6.

POINT 8 Is in the centre of the eyebrow directly above Point 5

POINT 9 Is slightly above the inner end of the eyebrow.

POINT 10 Is slightly below the inner end of the eyebrow.

Treatment of additional points

Hold machine in one hand, with your fingers on the steel plate and your thumb over the test/treat button (do not press yet) as shown in Figs 2 and 4 and slide tip over skin until you find the points detailed in pages 70-77. You should feel a stinging sensation, which is reduced by sliding the intensity switch down. Full instructions are included with the HealthPoint™ kit.

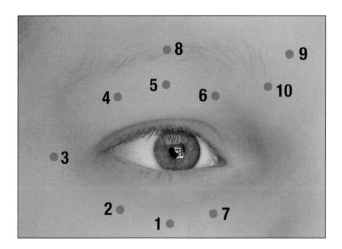

Fig. 1

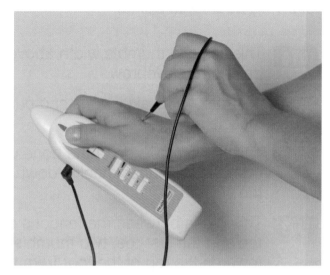

Fig. 2

The gold probe is used for the
additional points away from the eyes

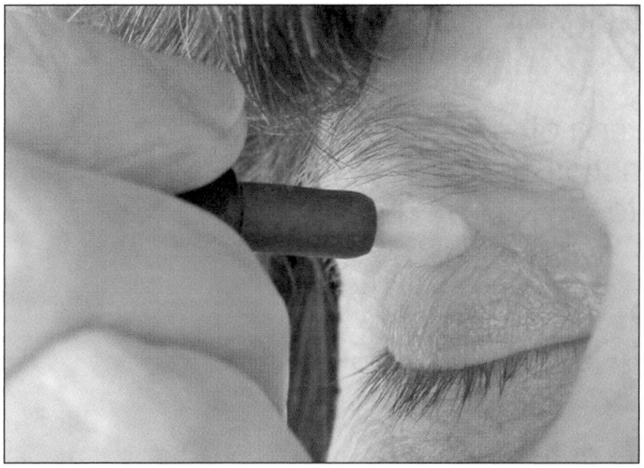

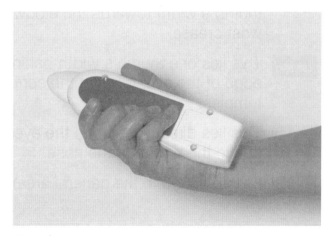

Fig. 3

Using the cotton bud probe as shown
here is the preferred method for
treating around the eyes

Fig. 4

MACULAR DEGENERATION or DIABETIC RETINOPATHY - EXTRA POINTS

First treat the Basic Points, then treat the following additional points:

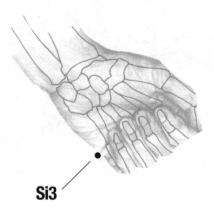

Si3

G14 This lies one thumb's width above the mid point of the eyebrow.

G20 Just below the skull bone and outside the muscle bulge.

Li4 This lies on the side of the bone which runs from the forefinger knuckle down towards the wrist.

Liv3 This lies in between the tendons of the big toe and the first toe, two thumb's width towards the top of the foot from the web.

S36 This lies three thumb's width below the joint under the kneecap lying on the outer side of the knee. One finger's width back from the sharp edge of the shin bone.

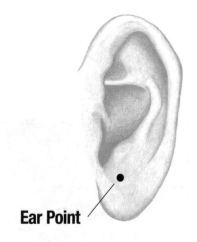

Ear Point

Si3 With the fist clenched, this lies at the end of the main crease of the palm at the junction of the red and white skin (It is easier to locate unclenched).

T5 This lies on the back of the wrist, two thumb's width towards the elbow from the wrist crease.

Taiyang This lies one thumb's width behind the outer edge of the eye. It lies in the centre of the temples.

Taiyang

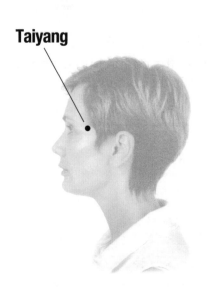

Yintang This lies directly between the eyebrows, just above the bridge of the nose.

Ear Ear point (2-3 in the general area)

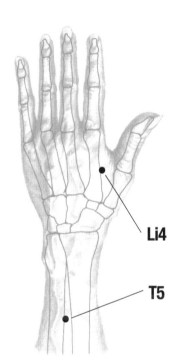

Yintang

G14

CATARACTS - EXTRA POINTS

*First treat the Basic Points, then treat the
following additional points:*

G14 This lies one thumb's width above the mid
point of the eyebrow.

Li4 This lies on the side of the bone which runs
from the forefinger knuckle down towards
the wrist.

Liv3 This lies in between the tendons of the big
toe and the first toe, two thumb's width
towards the top of the foot from the web.

S36 This lies three thumb's width below the joint
under the kneecap lying on the outer side of
the knee. One finger's width back from the
sharp edge of the shin bone.

Si3 With the fist clenched, this lies at the end of
the main crease of the palm at the junction
of the red and white skin (It is easier to
locate unclenched).

Ear Ear point (2-3 in the general area)

Li4

T5

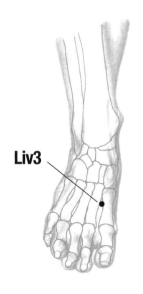

Liv3

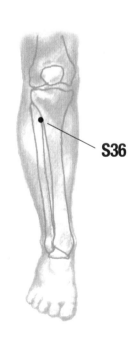

S36

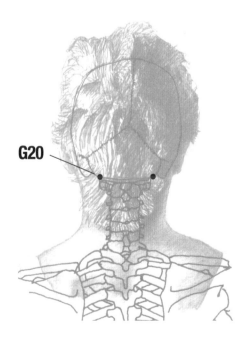

G20

CONJUNCTIVITIS - EXTRA POINTS

First treat the Basic Points, then treat the following additional points:

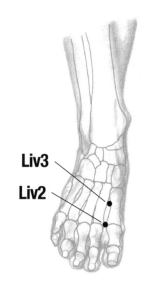

G14 This lies one thumb's width above the mid point of the eyebrow.

G20 Just below the skull bone and outside the muscle bulge.

Li4 This lies on the side of the bone which runs from the forefinger knuckle down towards the wrist.

Liv3 This lies in between the tendons of the big toe and the first toe, two thumb's width towards the top of the foot from the web.

S36 This lies three thumb's width below the joint under the kneecap lying on the outer side of the knee. One finger's width back from the sharp edge of the shin bone.

Yintang This lies directly between the eyebrows, just above the bridge of the nose.

Ear Ear point (2-3 in the general area)

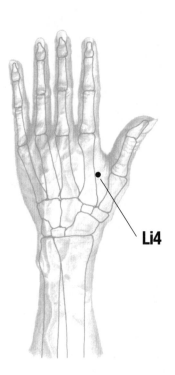

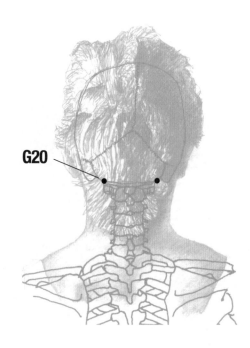

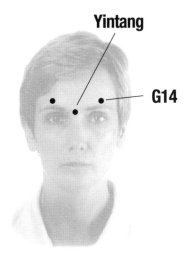

Yintang

G14

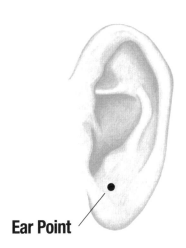

Ear Point

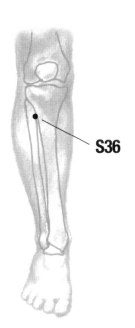

S36

GLAUCOMA - EXTRA POINTS

First treat the Basic Points, then treat the following additional points:

G20 Just below the skull bone and outside the muscle bulge.

K3 This lies midway between the tip of the inner ankle bone and the achilles tendon (in the hollow)

Li4 This lies on the side of the bone which runs from the forefinger knuckle down towards the wrist.

Liv2 This is one finger's width up from the web between the big toe and the second toe tendons.

Liv3 This lies in between the tendons of the big toe and the first toe, two thumb's width towards the top of the foot from the web.

S36 This lies three thumb's width below the joint under the kneecap lying on the outer side of the knee. One finger's width back from the sharp edge of the shin bone.

Sp6 This lies one hand's width (four fingers) up from the inner ankle joint. It lies just behind the tibia bone at this point.

Ear Ear point (2-3 in the general area)

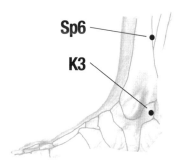

Sp6

K3

SQUINT - EXTRA POINTS

First treat the Basic Points, then treat the following additional points:

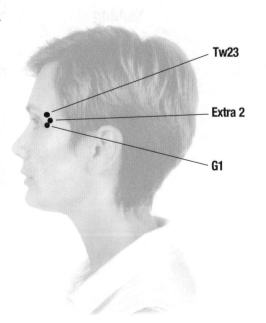

G1   This lies half a finger out from the outer corner of the eye

G20   Just below the skull bone and outside the muscle bulge.

Li4   This lies on the side of the bone which runs from the forefinger knuckle down towards the wrist.

Ear   Ear point (2-3 in the general area)

'MS' EYE PROBLEMS - EXTRA POINTS

First treat the Basic Points, then treat the following additional points:

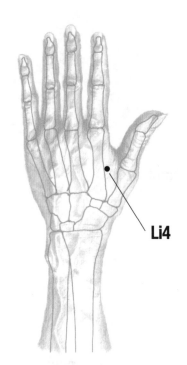

Extra 2   A finger behind a line drawn between the outer end of the eyebrow and the outer corner of the eye.

TW23   This is located at the outer end of the eyebrow.

Ear   Ear point (2-3 in the general area)

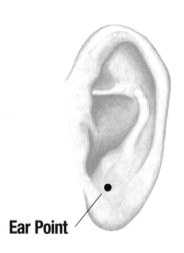

Ear Point

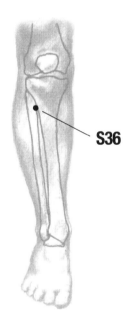

Yintang

G14

FLOATERS - EXTRA POINTS

First treat the Basic Points, then treat the following additional points:

G14 This lies one thumb's width above the mid point of the eyebrow.

G20 Just below the skull bone and outside the muscle bulge.

Li4 This lies on the side of the bone which runs from the forefinger knuckle down towards the wrist.

Liv3 This lies in between the tendons of the big toe and the first toe, two thumb's width towards the top of the foot from the web.

S36 This lies three thumb's width below the joint under the kneecap lying on the outer side of the knee. One finger's width back from the sharp edge of the shin bone.

Yintang This lies directly between the eyebrows, just above the bridge of the nose.

Ear Ear point (2-3 in the general area)

S36

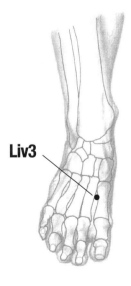

Liv3

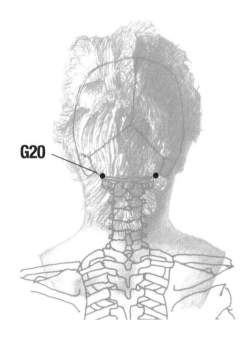

G20

COMPUTER EYE SYNDROME - EXTRA POINTS

First treat the Basic Points, then treat the following additional points:

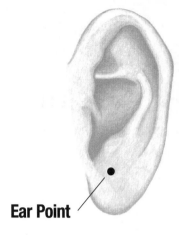

G14 This lies one thumb's width above the mid point of the eyebrow.

G20 Just below the skull bone and outside the muscle bulge.

Li4 This lies on the side of the bone which runs from the forefinger knuckle down towards the wrist.

Liv3 This lies in between the tendons of the big toe and the first toe, two thumb's width towards the top of the foot from the web.

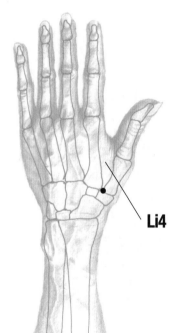

S36 This lies three thumb's width below the joint under the kneecap lying on the outer side of the knee. One finger's width back from the sharp edge of the shin bone.

Yintang This lies directly between the eyebrows, just above the bridge of the nose.

Ear Ear point (2-3 in the general area))

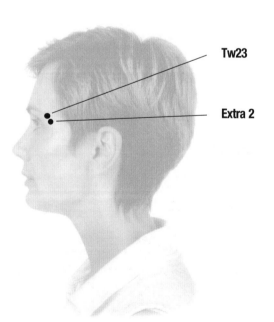

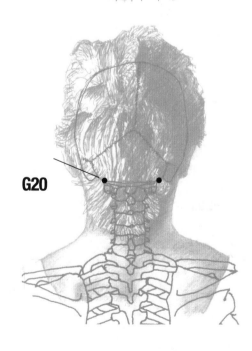

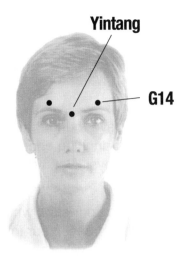

Yintang

G14

First treat the Basic Points, then treat the following additional points:

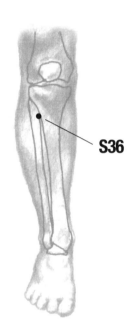

S36

G14 This lies one thumb's width above the mid point of the eyebrow.

G20 Just below the skull bone and outside the muscle bulge.

Li4 This lies on the side of the bone which runs from the forefinger knuckle down towards the wrist.

Liv3 This lies in between the tendons of the big toe and the first toe, two thumb's width towards the top of the foot from the web.

S36 This lies three thumb's width below the joint under the kneecap lying on the outer side of the knee. One finger's width back from the sharp edge of the shin bone.

Yintang This lies directly between the eyebrows, just above the bridge of the nose.

Extra 2 A finger behind a line drawn between the outer end of the eyebrow and the outer corner of the eye.

TW23 This is located at the outer end of the eyebrow.

Ear Ear point (2-3 in the general area))

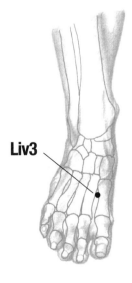

Liv3

3. WATER DATA SHEETS

I wrote earlier that water is one of the three essential components of maintaining life and good health. This is born out by the fact that you can only live a few days without water (or water-containing food).

I guarantee you are not drinking enough. Many natural health practitioners have found that a major part of the epidemic of degenerative diseases is dehydration from not drinking enough water. Water helps all the major organs to function more efficiently. The kidneys, liver, lymphatic system, arteries and veins all need adequate supplies of water to work at their optimum.

One of the most notable side effects of drinking 12 glasses of water a day is your skin, which is about 70% water. You will get complimented often on your skin when you increase your intake of water. Watch the cells plump up and wrinkles disappear... really! Headaches will also be reduced dramatically.

According to Dr. Susan Shireffs, of the Biomedical Services Department at Aberdeen University "By the time you are thirsty, you are already dehydrated. Even small levels of dehydration can cause headaches, lethargy, an overall lack of alertness and changes in mood."

So how can you tell if you are dehydrated? One way is by checking your urine. If it's bright yellow then you're probably dehydrated. Once you are rehydrated, it will become very pale and clear. Results, however, depend upon the quality of the water you consume. I'd suggest staying away from, or at least cutting down on, fizzy drinks. All those little bubbles are carbon dioxide, and I am sure we can all remember how photosynthesis works. We expel the carbon dioxide while breathing out, as it's poison to the body. So why do we choose to put it back in again in the form of carbonated drinks? Probably because we didn't know any better... but we do now!

Fizzy drinks like cola not only dehydrate you, but may also contain around eight cubes of sugar per can—even worse are the diet colas with huge amounts of chemicals like aspartame...UGH! Steer clear of these if you want good health.

We are walking around dehydrated... just think of a dried prune, and you've got the picture!

Muscles store about 16% of our water, so no wonder they are not able to function when dehydrated. They become flabby and soft and find it harder to hold the skeleton in its correct position. Once we have rehydrated our muscles, you may be surprised to see your posture change, as they are now able to hold the skeleton in place much more easily. This is where you often find that backache, and general aches and pains disappear.

The brain too, is mostly water, and dehydration shows as poor memory, inability to think quickly, and a general sluggish thought process. All of these symptoms are much improved by drinking lots more water—lots more than you think you need. Remember, we have to rehydrate first.

It's interesting to note that the Hypothalamus, the master of the endocrine system, houses both the receptors for thirst and hunger close together, so often these signals get confused. When we think we are hungry, we may in fact be thirsty and a glass of water will do the trick. The secret is not to wait until you feel thirsty, as by that point your body is telling you that you are already dehydrated.

You need to drink more water. Tea, coffee, juices, and specifically soft drinks, cannot be classified as water. Only water is water (and do not drink it regularly iced or chilled). The very best water in a clean natural environment is rainwater. If you have ever washed your hair in rainwater you will know what I mean. The other recommendations are listed below.

How Much to Drink? If you are not traveling and have regular access to the bathroom then the following is ideal:

❖ Drink 1 pint immediately on waking up in the morning. Do not eat or drink anything else for 30-60 minutes. If you are suffering from constipation (defined as less than 2 bowel movements per day) then make this 2 pints for a week and then try just 1 pint.

❖ Do not drink liquid with meals, as this will dilute your digestive juices. Then, to help your digestion even more, try to wait 30 minutes before you have a drink after your meal. The rest of the day drink 1 glass (1/2 pint) every waking hour until 7 pm. This should be 10-12 glasses per day, as well as the first pint. If you have bladder or prostate problems, this water is even more important and you should also call the "helpline" for the action plan to solve that problem urgently.

The best available water filter that can be plumbed in is the "Reverse Osmosis" filter. These also come as a counter-top unit and are the least difficult to look after. Reverse Osmosis filters range in price from around $250/ £160 for an under-sink version, to about $3000/£2000 for whole home water purification. (Call the help line, shown at the front of the book, for more info.)

Another good water filter is a water distiller. These come in two forms: the counter top, 1 gallon Distiller and a plumbed-in unit that fits in a cupboard. Both are only obtainable from specialist suppliers. They can be difficult to plumb in, and probably the counter top version, at about $300, is the best to start out with.

The next best filter is the carbon block filter or ceramic block filter. Both of these are normally plumbed-in but can come as "counter top" units that you fill up.

The most common of the "counter top" filters is the Jug filter that can be bought at most health stores or chemists. These are the best (except for determined health participants) and cost between $20-$30 each. I really do recommend that you start with one of these and move on to the other options when you have established your action plan for good health. The downside of it is that the filter needs changing every 2-4 weeks to remain effective. You can always keep this as a travel filter.

Unfortunately, most tap water does not meet EPA regulations and, even after using a water filter, traces of poisons such as aluminum, lead, cadmium, iron, arsenic and nitrates are still likely to be there. Anna Selby, the author of "H20: Healing Water for Mind and Body" states that about 800 chemicals have been found in drinking water.

The best way to filter your water is by fitting a filtering system that purifies your tap water and removes impurities including minerals, fluoride, e-coli bacteria and nitrates. A portable water filter does filter out the worst of the bacterial contaminants and is better than tap water—just remember to change the filter regularly.

When you are out traveling, bottled "still" water is acceptable as a temporary substitute. Important note—if your tap water comes from underground wells (water company or private), then you should seriously look at a good filter as the inorganic minerals can cause problems.

If you are determined to go with the tap water, then fill a jug with boiling water and leave it to stand for an hour before using it to allow the chlorine to evaporate. Try not to drink it from the tap.

4. FOODS & RECIPE DATA SHEETS

After taking a few extra nutrients, such as Lutein and Liquid Vitamins and Minerals, you will soon notice the difference in your eyes and how well you feel. Then you may be convinced that you need to look at your food to also help in your health recovery plan. What can you do?

There are a number of problems to overcome:

1. The fact is that the food we eat is low in the correct nutrients for your eye.

2. Even if you have enough, that nutrition may be blocked from being absorbed by eating too many starchy foods.

3. Your digestive system almost certainly does not function as well as it did when you were younger, which will stop absorption of the nutrients.

4. You are not getting enough digestive enzymes to digest and assimilate your food (remember a 70 year-old has only 20% of the enzymes compared to a 20 year-old).

5. Genetically, we may be incapable of absorbing the essential nutrients (which is why our plan works for those who have been told their problem is genetic).

What is the answer?

a. Low nutrient foods—all foods are now low in nutrients and this can only be solved by taking extra nutrition as detailed in this book. All nutrients detailed in this book have been proven in clinical use, as well as clinical studies. An example is Lutein Liposomal spray, which bypasses the digestive tract and enters the blood stream under the tongue, reaching the eyes within a few minutes. No matter how bad your digestive tract, Lutein spray will always be available to your eyes.

b. Grains, cereals, and other starchy foods, such as potatoes, are not natural healthy foods for humans (or animals). Eaten to excess, they have been proven in scientific studies to be a factor in poor health and the low uptake of nutrients. This also provides the perfect breeding ground for unfriendly bacteria and yeast in the intestines. As well as blocking nutritional uptake, damaging your eye cells through Glycation and replacing real food in your diet, they also cause the friendly bacteria that reside in your intestines to die off as the unfriendly bacteria increases. Friendly bacteria are called Probiotics, and they ensure that your intestines can deal with any food poisoning and manufacture B vitamins. They also help the uptake of various nutrients, especially the amino acid, Taurine, that are essential for healthy eyes and brain. You will need to reestablish your friendly flora, and you can read about this in the "Other Nutrients," Section 6. You will improve your chances of regaining your eyesight by cutting out all grains, cereals, potatoes, and other starchy foods for a few months, until you have recovered your health. Later, you can include a small amount of whole grains in your diet. I know this is the most difficult change covered in this book, but I cannot over-stress that the benefits will be worth it. You will lose all excess fat, start to build lean muscle, every part of your body will reverse its premature aging process, and you will feel more energetic.

c. Everyone is aware that their digestive system is the source of good health, yet very few people (or doctors) pay it much attention. A few tips are:

    a) Drink a small glass of Apple Cider vinegar before each meal to stimulate your digestive juices.

b) As well as cutting down on grains and cereals, cut down dairy products and meat (replace meat with various fish dishes)

c) Take Digestive Enzymes (see Other Nutrients in Section 6)

d) Do not drink liquid just before or after your meals.

e) Chew each mouthful of food at least 20 times (or blend if you have difficulty chewing).

f) Take longer to eat your meal, and eat only when relaxed.

g) Eat three meals every day, and only eat fruit between meals.

d. No food will be digested without Enzymes; no food will be assimilated without enzymes. Many natural practitioners just prescribe enzymes, water, and nutrition, and health recovery follows very quickly. If you cannot bear to eat your food raw, then you can only digest and assimilate it with additional enzymes taken before each meal.

e. When we eat a large amount of grains and cereals we do not realize we are missing out on foods that contain high levels of nutrients—there are very few nutrients (proportionately) in grains and cereals that are not found in real foods, as well as many more. What are real foods? Vegetables (mainly plants, with only a few root vegetables, as these may be high in starch), fruits, nuts, seeds, and beans. An example is the following list that shows the amount of Lutein per serving. There is none in grains and cereals.

Kale	21,900 mcg	Collard Greens	16,300 mcg
Spinach - cooked	12,600 mcg	Spinach - raw	10,200 mcg
Mustard Greens	9,900 mcg	Okra	6,800 mcg
Red Pepper	6,800 mcg	Romaine Lettuce	5,700 mcg
Endive	4,000 mcg	Cooked Broccoli	1,800 mcg
Green Peas	1,700 mcg	Pumpkin	1,500 mcg
Brussel Sprouts	1,300 mcg	Summer Squash	1,200 mcg

Include kale and a selection every day in your diet. See "Eyesight Soup" later in this section.

I explained earlier that excess glucose in the bloodstream causes Glycation. This is where the body's cells are damaged by this excess glucose and, unless you are a marathon runner, you will almost certainly be overdosing on glucose if you eat the standard amount of carbohydrates and starchy foods that has become the habit in the modern diet.

Where do we get this excess glucose? The foods that cause this unhealthy rise in glucose are called High Glycemic foods.

Glycemic Index

The Glycemic Index (G.I.) is a numerical system of measuring how fast a carbohydrate triggers a rise in circulating blood sugar—the higher the number, the greater the blood sugar response. So a low G.I. food will cause a small rise, while a high G.I. food will trigger a dramatic spike.

A list of carbohydrates with their Glycemic values is shown on the following pages. The list is ordered by the G.I., which makes it easy to locate high or low G.I. foods. Except as noted, each of the G.I. values shown is based on around 80 studies in the professional literature referenced in the G.I. Factor.

There are two Glycaemic indexes, based on:

1. White bread = 100 *or*
2. Glucose = 100.

The fact that there are two glycaemic indexes is confusing. I have shown the **Glucose Index.**

Scientists fed 50 grams of glucose to their test subjects. They saw that this amount of glucose raised their subjects' blood glucose to a certain level. They called that level 100, which became the base of the index. Then they tested their subjects with other foods. If, for example, one of those foods raised their test subjects' blood glucose level 70 percent as much on average as the glucose did, then they assigned an index of 70 to that food. And so on with other foods tested.

Try to substitute foods that are lower on the list for the higher Glycemic foods that you have been eating up till now. OBVIOUSLY, THE LOWER THE BETTER—in my opinion, less than 45 would be ideal.

DIABETES—By eating the low Glucose Index foods, you will also avoid or reverse Type 2, or age related diabetes.

Food Type	*Glycaemic Index*	*Warning*
Fruits Nopal prickly pear cactus	7	✔
Beans/Pulses/Grains Lentils, green, canned	8	✔
Beans/Pulses/Grains Soya beans, canned	14	✔
Yoghurt Sheep's milk	14	✔
Nuts Peanuts	15	*Contains Fungus* ✔
Beans/Pulses/Grains Soya beans	18	✔
Beans/Pulses/Grains Rajmah (red kidney beans)	19	✔
Rice Bran	19	✔
Eggs (Organic)	20	*Only naturally fed* ✔
Nuts Almonds	20	✔
Nuts Brazil Nuts	20	✔
Nuts Pine Kernels	20	✔
Nuts Walnuts	20	✔
Vegetables Alfalfa Sprouts Etc	20	✔
Vegetables Dandelion Leaves	20	✔
Vegetables Garlic	20	✔
Vegetables Kale	20	✔
Vegetables Lambs Lettuce	20	✔
Vegetables Mushrooms	20	✔
Vegetables Peas Mangtout	20	✔
Vegetables Peas Petit Pois	20	✔
Vegetables Peas Sugar-Snaps	20	✔
Fruits Cherries	22	✔
Vegetables Peas Dried	22	✔
Vegetables Seaweed (Wakame, Noni, Etc)	22	✔
Vegetables Fennel	23	✔
Sweets Milk, chocolate, artificially sweet	24	Never ✔
Vegetables Beans Runner	24	✔
Breads—Sprouted Bread (Sunnyvale)	25	✔
Bread – Sprouted Organic Wheat Grass Bread	25	✔

Fruits Bilberry	25		✔
Fruits Blackberry	25		✔
Fruits Grapefruit	25		✔
Fruits Nectarines	25		✔
Fruits Raspberries	25		✔
Fruits Rhubarb	25		✔
Quorn	25	*Not too much*	✔
Vegetables—Root Radish	25		✔
Vegetables Artichokes	25		✔
Vegetables Asparagus	25		✔
Vegetables Aubergines	25		✔
Vegetables Bamboo Sprouts	25		✔
Vegetables Broccoli	25		✔
Vegetables Brussels Sprouts	25		✔
Vegetables Cabbage Green	25		✔
Vegetables Cabbage Savoy	25		✔
Vegetables Cabbage White	25		✔
Vegetables Cauliflower	25		✔
Vegetables Celery	25		✔
Vegetables Chillies	25		✔
Vegetables Chinese Leaves	25		✔
Vegetables Chives	25		✔
Vegetables Courgettes	25		✔
Vegetables Cucumber	25		✔
Vegetables Curly Kale	25		✔
Vegetables Lettuce	25		✔
Vegetables Onions	25		✔
Vegetables Sorrel	25		✔
Vegetables Spinach	25		✔
Vegetables Spring Onion	25		✔
Vegetables Vine Leaves	25		✔
Vegetables Leeks	26		✔
Pasta Spelt Hemp oil enriched	27		✔
Vegetables Endives	27		✔
Vegetables Okra	27		✔
Fruits Strawberries	28	*Only in season*	✔
Quorn/Tofu Sausages	28	*Only occasionally*	✔
Beans/Pulses/Grains Kidney beans	29		✔
Gooseberries	29		✔
Beans/Pulses/Grains Spelt	30		✔
Bengal gram dal (chana dal)	30		✔
Breads Bürgen Oat Bran & Honey Loaf	30		✔
Cheese Feta (unpasterized)	30		✔
Cheese Goats (unpasterized)	30		✔
Fish Cod	30	*Not farmed*	✔
Fish Collee	30	*Not farmed*	✔
Fish eel	30	*Not farmed*	✔
Fish Haddock	30	*Not farmed*	✔
Fish Kippers	30	*Not farmed*	✔

Fish Mackerel	30	Not farmed	✔
Fish Plaice	30	Not farmed	✔
Fish Salmon (wild or Organic)	30	Not farmed	✔
Fish Sardines	30	Not farmed	✔
Fish Shellfish	30	Not farmed	✔
Fish Trout	30	Not farmed	✔
Fish Tuna	30	Not farmed	✔
Fruits Avocado	30		✔
Soy Products Soy Milk	30	Not babies	✔
Soy Products Tofu	30		✔
Vegetables Beans Mung	30		✔
Vegetables Peppers Red/Green/Yellow	30		✔
Fruits Dried Apricots, dried	31		✔
Beans/Pulses/Grains Lima beans, baby, frozen	32		✔
Beans/Pulses/Grains Millet	32		✔
Goats Milk, skimmed	32		✔
Spreads Chocolate spread	32	Occasionally	✔
Sweets Mars M&Ms (peanut)	32	Contains Fungus	✔
Vegetables Split peas, yellow, boiled	32		✔
Beans/Pulses/Grains Chick peas	33		✔
Yoghurt Goats milk	33		✔
Cheeky yam	34		✔
Sweets Milk, chocolate, sugar sweetened	34	Never Artificial	✔
Beans/Pulses/Grains Black beans	35		✔
Beans/Pulses/Grains Black Gram	35		✔
Beans/Pulses/Grains Black bean seed	35		✔
Beans/Pulses/Grains Black-eyed beans	35		✔
Beans/Pulses/Grains Broad beans	35		✔
Beans/Pulses/Grains Brown beans (Mexican)	35		✔
Beans/Pulses/Grains Brown beans	35		✔
Beans/Pulses/Grains Buckwheat	35		✔
Beans/Pulses/Grains Bulgur Wheat	35		✔
Beans/Pulses/Grains Butter beans	35		✔
Vegetables—Root Comfrey	35		✔
Vegetables—Root Kohlrabi	35		✔
Vegetables Beans French	35		✔
Vegetables Beans Green	35		✔
Vegetables Tomatoes	35		✔
Vegetables Water Chestnuts	35		✔
Vegetables Watercress	35		✔
Beans/Pulses/Grains Lima beans broth	36		✔
Yoghurt, unspecified	36		✔
Fruits Pear, fresh	37		✔
Pasta Spaghetti, wholemeal	37	Gluten and fungus	✔
Beans Baked (Whole Earth Organic, Sugar Free)	38		✔
Beans/Pulses/Grains Green gram (Mung beans)	38		✔
Beans/Pulses/Grains Haricot/Navy beans	38		✔
Fish fingers	38	Only occasional	✔

Food	Value	Note
Fruits Apple	38	✔
Soups Tomato Soup	38	✔
Soups Vegetables & Beans Homes Made	38	✔
Beans/Pulses/Grains Pinto beans	39	✔
Breads Barley kernel bread	39	✔
Fruits Plum	39	✔
Vegetable Marrowfat Peas, dried	39	✔
Fruits Damsons	40	✔
Fruits Dried Apple	40	✔
Fruits Dried Prunes	40	✔
Vegetables Baby Sweet corn Whole	40	✔
Vegetables Marrow	40	✔
Beans/Pulses/Grains Chick peas, curry, canned	41	✔
Fruits Juice Apple juice	41	✔
Beans/Pulses/Grains Chick peas, canned	42	✔
Breakfast Cereals All-bran	42	✔
Fruits Peach, fresh	42	✔
Bengal gram dal with semolina	43	✔
Breads Barley chapatti	43	✔
Puddings Custard	43	✔
Sweets Mars Twix Cookie Bars (caramel)	43	Occasional ✔
Fruits Orange	44	✔
Fruits Pear, canned	44	✔
Soups Lentil soup, canned	44	✔
Sweets Mars Chocolate	44	Occasional ✔
Vegetables—Root Sweet potato	44	✔
Vegetables—Root Turnip	44	✔
Beans/Pulses/Grains Pinto beans, canned	45	✔
Fruits Figs	45	✔
Yoghurt Yakult (fermented milk)	45	✔
Beans/Pulses/Grains Romano beans	46	?
Fruit Juices Pineapple juice	46	?
Fruits Grapes	46	?
Lactose	46	?
Soups Black bean soup	46	?
Fruits Peach, canned	47	?
Fruit Juices Grapefruit juice	48	?
Vegetables Peas, green	48	?
Breakfast Cereals Porridge (oatmeal)	49	?
Sweets Chocolate 30grams	49	Occasional ?
Vegetables - Root Carrots	49	?
Breads Pumpernickel	50	?
Puddings Ice cream, low fat	50	?
Horse gram	51	?
Vegetables Yam	51	?
Beans/Pulses/Grains Kidney beans, canned	52	?
Fruit Juices Orange juice	52	?
Fruits Kiwifruit	53	?

Beans/Pulses/Grains Lentils, red	54
Fruits Banana	54
Snacks Potatoes crisps	54
Vegetables—Root Swede	54
Biscuits Oatmeal cookies	55
Biscuits Rich Tea cookies	55
Cereal Sweetcorn	55
Fruits Fruit Cocktail (tin)	55
Rice Brown	55
Snacks Popcorn	55
Vegetables Sweet corn	55
Breakfast Cereals Muesli	56
Fruits Mango	56
Fruits Sultanas	56
Vegetables—Root Potatoes white	56
Breads Pita bread, white	57
Fruits Apricots, fresh	57
Rice Wild,	57
Vegetables—Root Potatoes new	57
Cereal Rice Basmati	58
Fruits Paw Paw	58
Rice Basmati rice	58
Rice Vermicelli	58
Rice White	58
Spreads Honey	58
Beans/Pulses/Grains Barley, cracked	60
Beans/Pulses/Grains Barley, pearled	60
Breads Pizza, cheese	60
Soups Split pea soup	60
Biscuits Muesli Bars	61
Breads Barm Cake bun	61
Sweets Mars Whole Grain Bars (choc chip)	61
Vegetables—Root Potatoes canned	61
Breads Maize chapatti	62
Green gram dal with semolina	62
Vegetables—Root Potatoes Prince Edward	63
Beans/Pulses/Grains Lentils, green	64
Biscuits Shortbread biscuits (2)	64
Breads Rye flour bread	64
Fruits Apricots, canned, syrup	64
Fruits Raisins	64
Pasta Macaroni and Cheese	64
Vegetables Beets	64
Beans/Pulses/Grains Couscous	65
Cereal Couscous	65
Fruits Melon (Cantaloupe, Honeydew, Galia)	65
Vegetables—Root Potatoes steamed	65
Beans/Pulses/Grains Barley, rolled	66

Drinks Cordial, orange	66
Fruits Pineapple	66
Soups Green pea soup, canned	66
Breads Croissant	67
Breakfast Cereals Grapenuts	67
Gnocchi	67
Breads Crumpet	69
Breads Ryvita	69
Breads Wholemeal	69
Breakfast Cereals Shredded Wheat	69
Beans/Pulses/Grains dried, P. Vulgaris	70
Breads Melba toast	70
Breads White	70
Breads White Bread (1 Slice)	70
Breakfast Cereals Weetabix (2)	70
Fruits Banana, unripe, steamed 1 hr.	70
Vegetables—Root Potatoes mashed	70
Biscuits Water Biscuits (5)	71
Breads Wheat bread, white	71
Breakfast Cereals Sultana Bran	71
Cereals Millet	71
Breads Bagel, white	72
Fruits Watermelon	72
Vegetables—Root Swede	72
Vegetables—Root Potatoes boiled, mashed	73
Breads Bread Stuffing	74
Breads Whole-wheat bread	74
Breakfast Cereals Cheerios	74
Breakfast Cereals Puffed Wheat	74
Snacks Corn chips	74
Corn Bran	75
Vegetables—Root Potatoes Chips (French Fries)	75
Vegetables Pumpkin	75
Breakfast bars	76
Breakfast Cereals Waffles	76
Cakes Donut	76
Biscuits Vanilla Wafer Biscuits (6)	77
Breakfast Cereals Coco pops	77
Jowar	77
Rice Cakes	77
Breads Wheat bread, Wonder white	78
Green gram dal + paspalum scorbic.	78
Biscuits Morning Coffee cookies	79
Sweets Jelly beans	80
Breads Puffed Crispbread	81
Puddings Tapioca, boiled with milk	81
Snacks Pretzels	81
Breakfast Cereals Rice Krispies	82

Vegetables—Root Potatoes microwaved	82	X
Breakfast Cereals Cornflakes	83	X
Vegetables—Root Potatoes instant	83	X
Vegetables—Root Potatoes baked	85	X
Breads, gluten free	90	X
Breads Wheat bread, gluten free	90	X
Rice Bubbles	90	X
Rice Instant, boiled 6 min	90	X
Spreads Jams and marmalades	91	X
Rice Pasta, brown	92	X
Breads French baguette	95	X
Drinks Lucozade	95	X
Drinks Glucose	96	X
Vegetables - Root Parsnips	97	X
Glucose tablets	102	X
Fruits Dates	103	X
Maltodextrin	105	X
Maltose	105	X
Puddings Tofu frozen desert, non-dairy	115	X
Tofu Ice cream	123	X

Meal Ideas

Examples of recipes that include really high nutrient food, with low Glycemic numbers are at the end of this section.

Important Note: Do not microwave your food nor overheat. This will kill the enzymes that are vital for your good health.

Breakfast Ideas

❖ EyeSight Soup™ (See recipe later)

❖ Organic Eggs—Boiled, Poached (on spinach) Scrambled, with tomatoes, mushrooms and/or vegetable omelettes (no cheese).

❖ Occasional Porridge with Soya or skimmed Milk.

❖ Fresh Fruit salad—with Soya yogurt etc. (check previous table for low glycaemic fruits)

❖ Kippers and Tomatoes

Replace flour bread with Sprouted Wheat bread. This is a healthy bread described in the Old Testament and consists of 100% organic sprouted grains (see data sheet later).

Lunch Ideas

❖ EyeSight Soup™ (at least once per day)

❖ Salads—Greek Salad, Avocado Salad, Salad Nicoise (no potatoes), Fish salad (Tuna, Herring, Salmon, Pilchards, or Sardines), or 3 Bean Salad. (Note: do not fill up on lettuce, consider instead, red/green/yellow peppers, onions, tomatoes, garlic, etc.).

❖ Sugar free, organic baked beans, mushrooms and tomatoes etc.

❖ Raw veggie sticks with hummous or similar.

❖ Leftover food from previous night.

Evening Meal Ideas

❖ Vegetables—Stir-fried, Steamed, Flash Boiled, Oven Roasted in olive oil.

❖ Tofu Chunks once or twice per week.

❖ Add Fish (oily fish Salmon (not farmed unless organic), Sardines, Mackerel, Trout and Eel at least 3-4 times per week) in place of meat. Haddock and Cod etc. do not contain high enough levels of EPA and DHA to count.

❖ Meat once or twice per week.

❖ Potatoes once per week.

❖ Baked sweet potatoes twice per week.

❖ Vegetable Curry with Bean curry (Chickpea Dahl) etc. (if absolutely necessary, include very small amount of rice).

❖ Vegetable Chilli.

❖ Fish and Vegetable Stew.

Eat 1 piece of low-sugar fruit between meals (mid-morning, mid-afternoon and mid-evening).

A delicious healthy snack or replacement for cake is Fruit Sprouted Wheat Bread (see data sheet later). Also, a bar of chocolate or chocolate raisins/nuts are a reasonably healthy snack.

Recipes

EyeSight Soup

Eat it most days at breakfast, lunch or evening meal.

Make enough to last for 3-4 days if you have room to keep it in the fridge. One idea is to put each day's soup into plastic containers, which may fit more easily into the fridge.

Vegetable Ideas (Choose 5-6 vegetables, only include 1-2 root vegetables).

Kale (important)	Sea Weed (Noni, Kelp, Wakame etc.)
Carrots	Purple broccoli
Peas	Spinach
Broccoli	Cabbage
Green beans	Brussels Sprouts
Spring greens	Cauliflower
Asparagus	Water Cress
Red & Yellow Peppers	

Plus

Onions (lots of)

Celery

Tinned Tomatoes

Garlic

Tinned Beans *(Choose 2-3 types, e.g Haricot, Soya beans, kidney beans, Chickpeas, Ballotti, Lentils, Black Eyed beans. (all tinned, sugar free, ready to use or dried and cook your own)* etc.

Plus

Rock Salt or Celtic Sea Salt

Vegetable Stock Cube

Seasoning

Oil

Cooking

1. Put 2 tablespoons of oil in a large pan, chop onion, carrots and celery. Cook for approximately 5 minutes.

2. Add rest of chopped vegetables, tinned tomatoes and boiling water plus the vegetable stock cube and minced garlic.

3. Simmer for 5-10 minutes, until just cooked.

4. Remove from heat and then blend to suit your taste.

5. Return to pan and add pulses and beans.

6. Allow to cool and refrigerate in containers or pan.

Make enough to last 4-5 days if kept in fridge. It can be frozen, if necessary.

Fish and Vegetable Stew

Eat it 1-3 times per week with different fish.

Make enough to last for 1 -2 meals, if you have room to keep it in the fridge (or longer in freezer). One idea is to put each day's meal into plastic containers, which may fit more easily into the fridge.

Ingredients suggestions:

Kale (important)	Sea Weed (Noni, Kelp, Wakame etc.)
Green beans	Broccoli
Sweet Potato	Red & Yellow Peppers
Spinach	Cabbage
Muscles	Salmon (not fish-farmed)
Coley	Sole
Prawns	Mackerel
Clams	Any fish to taste

Plus

Rock Salt

Garlic

Tinned Tomatoes

Tomato Puree

Red Onions

Seasoning

Sunflower Oil

Cooking

1. Heat 2 tablespoons of oil in a large pan.

2. Fry onions for 2 minutes then take onion out leaving oil in.

3. Add diced fish to the oil and fry on high heat for 2 minutes to seal the fish.

4. Add the cooked onion and then the rest of the chopped vegetables.

5. Add Tomatoes, seasoning, minced garlic and stock (water) to taste.

6. Bring to boil, then reduce heat to gently simmer for 20-30 minutes.

7. Add any prawns or shellfish 5 minutes before end. (you can keep all of the previously cooked fish out until this point if you prefer chunkier pieces.)

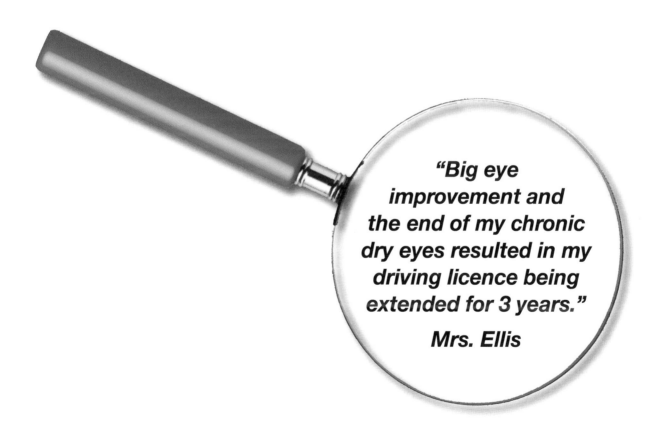

"Big eye improvement and the end of my chronic dry eyes resulted in my driving licence being extended for 3 years."

Mrs. Ellis

5. OXYGEN AND EXERCISE DATA SHEETS

The most important element of life is Oxygen.

Eighty percent of all the energy in the body comes from oxygen, with the remaining 20% coming from fats and glucose. Just a few minutes without it means certain death or brain damage. A shortage of oxygen in our cells means we do not have enough physical and mental energy, (your brain takes 25% of all the available oxygen), our cells would not have enough energy to regenerate properly, and we leave ourselves open to infections and cancer.

Oxygen does a fabulous job—when we get enough of it. Although it is very volatile and can (metaphorically) set our body on fire with free radicals, as long as we eat lots of vegetables and fruit that contain the famous antioxidants, everything can work in harmony.

Why do we not get enough Oxygen?

- Poor Breathing
- Sedentary Life
- Pollution
- Emotional stress or possibly from trauma
- Infections.

In a nutshell:

- If we do not have enough oxygen in our body we degenerate rapidly.
- If we do not have enough vegetables and fruits in our diet to provide antioxidants to keep the oxygen-free radicals in check, we can degenerate rapidly.

The answer is simple, get more oxygen and eat more fruit and vegetable.

How do we get more Oxygen?

There are two things we need to do to improve our available oxygen to our cells.

1. Breathing better

It seems so simple, but the fact remains that you almost certainly breathe from your chest instead of from your diaphragm. Those of you who have had singing training will know immediately what I am talking about. If I asked you to take a deep breath many people would immediately fill their chests with air and shoulders would rise. This is the wrong way to get more air into your body. The way to practice correct breathing is to take a deep breath and fill your diaphragm (or tummy) and then fill your chest. Hold this for the count of four and then exhale pulling your tummy in and underneath your rib cage. Hold it there for the count of four and then inhale.

You would take in 3 times more air (and three times more oxygen) than breathing into your chest and get a better balance of carbon dioxide. "Does it matter?" I hear you say. Well yes; if you breathe into your chest, then your body will consider this to be a signal that you are under stress and put your body into a stress mode. This mode includes closing down your capillaries (making your limbs colder), closing down your digestive system and upsetting your hormones.

What went wrong with breathing?

The main reason we start to breathe into our chest is because we allow our stomach muscles to become flabby and, particularly, the inside set of muscles that are essential for breathing out—or we were stressed for so long we forgot how to relax. If you do not breathe out fully by pulling your stomach in and up underneath your rib cage then of course you cannot get new air into your lungs. It could be said specifically "that breathing out is more important than breathing in."

Practice your new breathing lying down first on your back, with your hands on your stomach level with your navel, and feel them rise and fall as you breathe.

2. Aerobic Exercise

The second and equally important way of improving oxygen availability is to exercise aerobically. That is, just enough to get our heart beating and our lungs working. Oxygen is needed to help regenerate your cells in your eyes and the rest of your body. It is also needed as the main tool of your immune system to fight germs. Do this by building up to 15 minutes, twice a day initially for a month and then 30 minutes daily for another month, and finally 45 minutes. When you exercise, do not sit down until your time is complete, even if you cannot exercise all of the time. This stops you from cutting your exercise time too easily.

Which exercise is best?

You chose what is good for you, but whatever you choose to be sure to elevate your heart rate and be active for one hour every day. Your ideal exercise should elevate your heart rate to 180 beats per minute less than your age. For example, a person of 60-years-old would have a heart rate of 120 beats per minute (180-60=120). Remember that it is important to keep that going for one hour every day. If you do not want to buy a heart rate monitor to measure your level of exercise, then you should exercise just enough to make it feel slightly uncomfortable. This is not the best way and you should really put a heart-rate monitor on your birthday present list.

The Best— Walking fast for 1 hour every day is the very best exercise that anyone can do. Your arms should be swinging and you should stride out as far as you can. This gets your lymphatic system working to get rid of toxins in your body. Your diaphragm and breathing will start to work in harmony, and this exercise will also strengthen your muscles. Dancing is, of course, a wonderful additional "fun exercise," but remember it is "additional."

2nd Best— Rebounding on a 3' wide mini trampoline with a built in handrail to keep you steady. When you get stronger you can start to move your arms and legs.

3rd Best— Running on the spot and all the exercises that you did at school, e.g., jumping jacks and arm exercises.

4th Best— Swimming fast enough to make you breathless. I see many elderly people swimming breaststroke, up and down the pool, in a leisurely manner; and they think they are exercising. When they get out, they are never out of breath. What use is that? If you are not breathless, then you are not getting any extra oxygen into your body, and that is the whole point of aerobic exercise.

Note: You chose what is good for you, but whatever you choose to be sure to elevate your heart rate and be active for one hour every day. Your ideal exercise should elevate your heart rate to 180 beats per minute less than your age. For example, a person of 60-years-old would have a heart rate of 120 beats per minute (180-60=120). Remember that it is important to keep that going for one hour every day. Heart attacks are the most common reason for premature death.

What if I cannot exercise or I am immobile?

In the case of a person who has a genuine reason as to why they cannot exercise, then there are oxygen supplements that can be taken.

1. OxySorb— An enzyme derived from Seaweed that improves cell respiration and oxygen absorbance.

This is a nutritional supplement that has been the subject of many studies showing that it improves the oxygen level in the body. It is used by air travellers, flight crews, and athletic men and women. Sufferers of lung problems, such as emphysema, benefit by being able to give up their oxygen bottle.

While I really do recommend that exercise is the better way to improve the oxygen levels in the blood, if you cannot exercise then you must improve the oxygen by another method. OxySorb is a good and easy way to get that oxygen. You can read all about it in the "Other Nutrients" data sheets on the following pages.

2. Oxygen Drops – From stabilized double buffered oxygen.

These are taken in a glass of water and release oxygen into the intestines and eventually into the body.

Dynamo2 is the ONLY "stabilized oxygen" product that is DOUBLE buffered to continuously release its oxygen both in the acid environment of the stomach, and in the alkaline environment of the intestines—for improved intestinal functioning. Also offered enhanced with MSM to provide bio-available sulphur at the cellular level, to enhance immunity in the intestines. This is used worldwide, with over 1,000,000 servings sold.

Which should you take?

Try the first, and if you do not feel any great benefit, then try the second. Either way, you can get more oxygen in your body.

"My eyes seem much better after only 2 months, although some days are better than others. The TV seems much clearer."

Mrs. Connolly

6. OTHER NUTRIENTS DATA SHEETS
Probiotic14™

Supplement Facts:

120 Veggie Capsules per bottle

Activity per capsule:

Probiotic Blend 1,200,000,000 CFU*

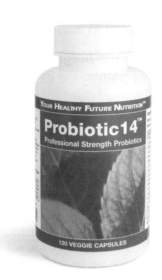

Lactobacillus acidophilus	600,000,000 CFU
Lactobacillus plantarum	600,000,000 CFU
Bifidobacterium longum	600,000,000 CFU
Bifidobacterium infantis	600,000,000 CFU
Lactobacillus bulgaricus	600,000,000 CFU
Streptococcus thermophilus	600,000,000 CFU
Lactobacillus casei	600,000,000 CFU
Lactobacillus salivarius	600,000,000 CFU
Bifidobacterium breve	600,000,000 CFU
Lactobacillus paracasei	600,000,000 CFU
Lactobacillus rhamnosus	600,000,000 CFU
Lactobacillus lactis	600,000,000 CFU
Lactobacillus brevis	600,000,000 CFU
Fructooligosaccharides	200mg

CFU - Colony Forming Units

Directions: As a nutritional supplement, take 2 capsules immediately on rising and 2 capsules at bedtime, or as directed by your healthcare professional.

Benefits:

- ❖ Helps avoid Food allergies
- ❖ Helps with Diarrhoea
- ❖ Helps Prevent Herpes
- ❖ Helps Prevent Cold
- ❖ Helps Prevent Viral Infections
- ❖ Helps Prevent Food Poisoning
- ❖ Helps with Chronic constipation
- ❖ Helps with Chronic Fatigue Syndrome
- ❖ Helps Prevent Epstein Barr Virus
- ❖ Helps Prevent 'Flu'
- ❖ Helps Prevent Parasites
- ❖ Helps Prevent Fungus
- ❖ Improves uptake of Taurine (for eyes and brain)

Probiotic14™ plays a critical role in digesting undigested protein and other foods.

Lactobacillus acidophilus is a normal inhabitant of the intestinal tract and the most numerous of the lactobacilli. It is considered to be the most beneficial lactobacillus in the intestine. Some of the beneficial effects attributed to Lactobacillus acidophilus are: cholesterol reduction, inhibition of undesirable bacteria, improved lactose intolerance, reduced carcinogen production, and improved immune response. This bacterium is also the predominant bacteria in the normal flora of the vagina, where it has a role in inhibiting infections.

Bifidobacterium bifidum is the natural component in the small intestine and is the predominant bacteria in the intestine of breast-fed infants. It is also part of the intestinal bacteria in adults. It produces acetic and lactic acid and may keep the pH low in the small intestine, which inhibits E.Coli. Often added as a Probiotic to milk or yogurt.

Bifidobacterium infantis is similar to Bifidobacterium bifidum, flourishes in breast-fed infants and is not usually found in adults. It manufactures B-vitamins, and may detoxify the intestines. Useful for children with food allergies.

Bifidobacterium longum stimulates the immune system by enhancing the activity of natural killer cells in the spleen. The mechanisms of immune support by Bifidobacterium longum have been studied in animals.

Lactobacillus bulgaricus is a high producer of Lactase which digests sugars in dairy products. Destroys pathogens in large intestine when introduced. May help alleviate painful arthritis.

Lactobacillus plantarum aids in the balance of beneficial bacteria in the large intestine and produces lactic acid that is vital to balancing the pH in the colon. It inhibits the translocation of bacteria from the gut to other organs such as lymph nodes and liver.

Intestinal toxicity leads to a low immune system. Accumulation of toxins in the colon diverticula causes Diverticulitis and other problems. L. Plantarum can be utilized throughout the whole gastrointestinal track, eliminating toxins and balancing the environment. The colonies continue to grow and produce a natural antibiotic effect, aiding the immune system in its fight against harmful agents in the body.

Streptococcus thermophilus is a good source of lactase to aid digestion of milk sugar.

Lactobacillus casei is an inhabitant of the intestinal tract and has been demonstrated to have an immunostimulatory effect by the intestinal secretion of IgA and thus promoting the gut immune barrier. May reduce the severity of diarrhoea in children.

Lactobacillus salivarius has been proven to be capable of producing a high amount of lactic acid and could inhibit and reduce the inflammatory response of H.pylori. Fructooligosaccharides (FOS) is an effective nutrient for intestinal Probiotic bacteria. The Probiotics have to have some good flora to enable them to work. Normal human enzymes cannot digest FOS, which allows it to enter the colon intact and become a nutrient for the good bacteria.

See the resources page at the end for supplier details

Liver Balance Plus™

The health of your liver is closely linked to the health of your eyes and an unhealthy liver will quickly be reflected in the whites of your eyes and blurred vision. For example, excess alcohol damages the liver and you will notice that drunken people always screw their eyes up. The liver is responsible for processing and removing toxins from your body, converting beta carotene to Vitamin A, storing vitamins and much more. Liver Balance Plus™ provides a rich blend of herbs with a long tradition of supporting this major organ:

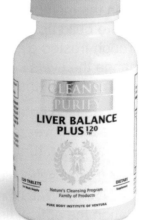

Proprietary Blend of:

- Dong Quai Root
- Dandelion Root
- Peony Root
- Poria
- Cocos Root
- Chinese Mint Leaf
- Cayenne Leaf
- Bupleurum Root
- Tribulus Terrestris
- Atractylodes Root
- Ginger Root
- Licorice Root
- Hyssop Leaf
- Chamaelirum Luteum Root

Suggested Dosage:

By symptom: Take 5 tablets when you have a liver symptom. Initially, this could be several times a day.

Intensive: Every 2 hours take 3-5 tablets. Cut off time is 7:00pm.

Please note: Always skip one day a week, can be take with or without food.

See the resources page at the end for supplier details

MSM+Silver™ Water Drops

Your eye is like a water balloon. The optical tissue normally allows fluids to flow through the membrane wall, which acts like a filter, supplying nutrition and cleaning out particles, keeping your eye clear so your vision is good.

When the membranes become tough like leather, fluids are trapped, and particles start to build up. If the build up continues, it will seem as if you are looking through frosted glass. Our eyes should also be flexible, so the muscles can change the eye's contour and focus. When the eye membranes and muscles become tough, the eye cannot focus properly and vision becomes blurry.

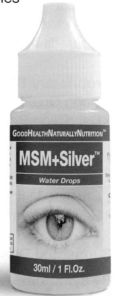

When treating irritated eyes, most eye drops and medications deaden the nerves and cover the pain, but the problem is not solved and the discomfort returns. We, in turn, buy more eye drops to relieve the discomfort.

MSM (Methylsulfonylmethane) is natural sulphur that resides in the body. MSM+Silver Water Drops soften the membranes, allowing fluids to pass through the optical tissues.

When our optical membranes become permeable, nutrients are able to penetrate through the optical tissues and provide nutrients needed for the body to heal itself. MSM softens tough, leathery tissue, equalizes pressure, repairs damaged membranes, clears up red spots and broken blood vessels, and helps remove floaters and other eye particles.

Colloidal Silver is an amazing alternative to Antibiotics. Biomedical research has shown that Colloidal Silver can help combat bacteria, virus or fungal infections. Also resistant strains fail to develop when using silver as a treatment plus at the correct concentration it is virtually non-toxic to humans.

Related Diseases to be helped:

Blepharitis, Computer Vision Syndrome, Conjunctivitis, Dry Eyes, Floaters, Glaucoma, Iritis, Kerataconus and Pterygium.

See the resources page at the end for supplier details

Essential Digestive Plus™

An example of a minimum formula; Plant enzyme activity (per capsules):

FrutaFit®IQ Inulin	150mg
Protease SP Blend	82,000 HUT
Amylase	8.000 DU
Alpha-Galactosidase	300 GLA
Glucoamylase	20 AGU
Lactase	1,0000 ALU
Cellulase	600 CU
Invertase	525 INVU
Pectinase	55 endo PGU
Lipase	1350 FIPL

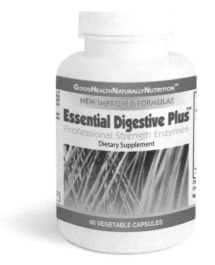

Directions:

Take 1 Capsule before each meal, or as directed by a health professional

Children and pets may use Essential Digestive Plus™ under supervision. If there is any difficulty in swallowing the capsules, open them and mix the powder with the food. Essential Digestive Plus™ taken between meals may be beneficial in cases of food allergies, toxicity, and drug withdrawal.

- ❖ Supports friendly bacteria
- ❖ Helps prevent indigestion
- ❖ Helps avoid Mal-absorption
- ❖ Helps avoid Gastritis
- ❖ Helps avoid Hiatus Hernia

- ❖ Helps avoid Food allergies
- ❖ Helps avoid Gallbladder stress
- ❖ Helps avoid Intestinal toxemia
- ❖ Helps avoid Gastric or Duodenal Ulcers
- ❖ Helps avoid Constipation

Constipation

1. Cut down or cut out all bread, pastry, grains, cereals etc.
2. Drink 1-2 pints of water immediately on waking. Then wait 1 hour before eating breakfast.
3. Drink 1 glass of water every hour during the day.
4. Increase vegetables and fruit to 8 portions of vegetable and 3 fruit per day. Make homemade vegetable soup in large pan to last a few days. Include cabbage in the soup.
5. Walk very fast for 30-45 minutes every day.

See the resources page at the end for supplier details

Organic Sprouted Wheat Bread

Centuries ago, especially in biblical times, bread was made simply, purely and naturally, using just sprouted wheat and water. This is believed to be the healthiest of bread. Now such bread is available again, but this time with a number of varieties to choose from. ORGANIC SPROUTED BREAD is available in Original Plain, or with Raisins, Dates and Fruit and Almond.

Benefits:

- ❖ Sprouted grain bread has almost double the fibre and protein content, than any other bread

- ❖ It is lower in calories, and virtually fat and salt free.

- ❖ It is ideal for people looking for a low fat, energy food, as it provides sustained energy using complex carbohydrates.

- ❖ It is also ideal for an increasing number of people with special dietary needs as it contains no ingredients other than Organic Wheat Grass and filtered water—no flour, yeast, fats, sugar, sweeteners, eggs, salt or dairy products.

- ❖ Sprouted Wheat breads have been known to be eaten by those on Wheat-Free, and Gluten-Free diets as well, with no detrimental effects.

- ❖ But perhaps most remarkably, despite its healthy ingredients, it is delicious too!

The high nutritional content of the sprouted grain bread is achieved through the special process by which it is made.

1. Firstly, they soak only the best Organic wheat kernels in pure filtered water, under tightly controlled conditions.

2. These are then allowed to sprout naturally. Once full germinated, the sprouts are ground, blended with organic dried fruit where appropriate, formed into loaf shapes and baked slowly and gently at low temperatures. Sprouting of the grain significantly increases the protein, vitamin and enzyme content of the breads, while complex starches in the grain are converted to natural sugars, providing the body with an easily digested, rich energy source.

Because the whole grain is used, the breads contain 100% of the bran fiber and wheat germ of the original grain, naturally producing typically almost double the fiber content of everyday bread. The resulting bread is highly nutritious, traditional, filling, as well as full of flavor.

Eat Right for Your Type: Research in the USA by Dr. D'Adamo has shown that to maintain perfect health, we should eat according to our blood type, because the different lectins in food react differently in our bodies, that is, your blood type determines which foods are right for you. This research has also shown that though wheat is not suitable for all blood types, sprouted wheat, on the other hand, is suitable for ALL blood types.

As if all of the above was not enough, the Original Sprouted Bread is also available in the following delicious Flavors: Raisin, Date and Fruit & Almond.

Organic sprouted wheat breads are available in most good health stores, but in case of difficulty, please call the help line, shown at the front of the book to find your nearest location.

General Information

❖ Vitamin 'E' is recommended at high doses, but build up slowly to 1200iu per day.

❖ Gingko is not absolutely necessary, if you are taking the Lutein Spray; but if you prefer to take it, then it is fine to do so.

❖ Bilberry is especially good, if you have leaky capillaries etc.

❖ Lycopene is a recommended extra nutrient for the eyes and protection against cancer.

❖ Probiotic friendly bacteria is important for general health, as well as making sure that Taurine is absorbed properly. Taurine for healthy eyes and brain.

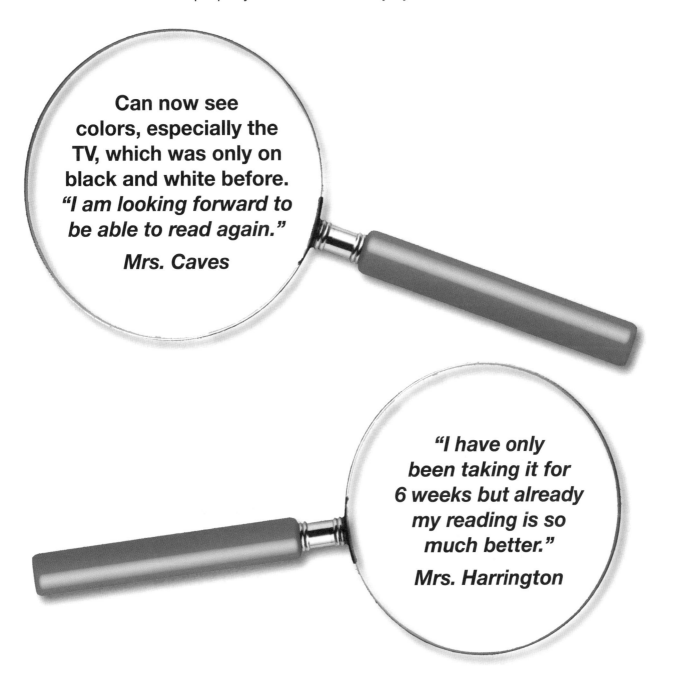

Can now see colors, especially the TV, which was only on black and white before. *"I am looking forward to be able to read again."*

Mrs. Caves

"I have only been taking it for 6 weeks but already my reading is so much better."

Mrs. Harrington

Curcumin98™—the most important Herb?

Turmeric has long been revered as the foundation of an herbal program for health. In Ayurvedic medicine, it has been recognized for thousands of years as a key balancing and detoxifying herb and is considered to be one of the very best all-round herbs for general well-being.

Curcumin is the main biologically active part of Turmeric, which only contains 4% Curcumin, whereas Curcumin98™ contains 98%. It has been identified in pharmacology as: anti-bacterial, anti-viral, anti-fungal, anti-yeast, anti-allergenic, anti-inflammatory, anti-oxidant, anti-spasmodic, carminative, diuretic, and anti-tumor.

Curcumin Treating eye disorders

Curcumin is, apparently, more than your typical kitchen spice. It has been implicated in the treatment of certain eye diseases and conditions. One of those is known as chronic anterior uveitis (CAD), an inflammatory condition of the vascular layer of the eye, particularly the area comprising the iris. In one small study, Curcumin was given orally to 32 CAD patients who were divided into two groups. The first group received Curcumin alone, whereas the second group received a combination of Curcumin and antitubercular treatment. Amazingly, all of the patients treated with Curcumin alone improved, compared to a response rate of 86% among those receiving the combination therapy. The researchers concluded that Curcumin was just as effective as corticosteroid therapy, the only available standard treatment for chronic anterior uveitis at present, adding that "the lack of side effects with Curcumin is its greatest advantage compared with corticosteroids."

Similar research using rats and rabbits found that Curcumin effectively inhibited chemically induced cataract formation, even at very low dietary levels. In one of the earliest studies examining Curcumin as a potential cataract therapy, researchers fed two groups of rats, diets that included corn oil, or a combination of Curcumin and corn oil, for 14 days. Afterward, their lenses were removed and examined for the presence of lipid peroxidation. The scientists discovered that "the lenses from Curcumin-treated rats were much more resistant to induced opacification than were lenses from control animals."

Awasthi S et al. Curcumin protects against 4-hydroxy-2-trans-nonenal-induced cataract formation in rat lenses. Am J Clin Nutr 1996 Nov;64 (5):761-6.

Lai B et al. Efficacy of curcumin in the management of chronic anterior uveitis. Phytother Res 1999 Jun;13(4):318-22.

Pandya U et al. Dietary curcumin prevents ocular toxicity of naphthalene in rats. Toxicol Lett 2000 Jun 5; 115(3): 195-204.

www.curcuminhealth.info

Contents: 180 Veggie Capsules each containing 400mg (total 72.000mg)

N-Acetyl Carnosine Eye Drops

N-Acetyl Carnosine Eye Drops, (MAC drops) have been developed by a joint Russian-American team of scientists and are being heralded as a breakthrough in the treatment of cataracts.

The statistics in the human trials show that N-acetyl carnosine eye-drops applied for 6 months, (twice daily into the eye) had the following results:

88.9% had an improvement of glare sensitivity.

41.5% had an improvement of the transmissivity of the lens.

90% had an improvement in visual acuity.

In addition to cataracts, N-Acetyl Carnosine eye drops are also a lubricant and have been found to benefit

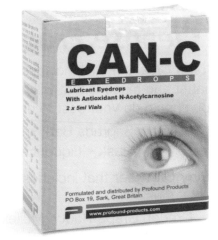

- ❖ Contact lens irritation
- ❖ Eye strain
- ❖ Blurred vision
- ❖ Night vision syndrome
- ❖ Computer vision syndrome
- ❖ Irritation and burning
- ❖ Dry eye syndrome
- ❖ Retinal diseases

N.B. It is important to ensure that you purchase only the N-Acetyl Carnosine eye drops that were used in the studies, as these are the only ones that have proven results. A number of copies have been marketed, some with added vitamin A, which may not have the level of purity required to treat the eyes safely.

Use 2 drops per eye, twice a day. It is important to keep up the treatment, which will take several months.

N-Acetyl Carnosine eye-drops should be used in addition to Lutein formula sublingual spray, not in place of it.

7. HERBAL CLEANSE DATA SHEETS

Before I list the various herbal cleanse and liver supports, I must stress that drinking more water is even more essential when taking herbs. The herbs' detoxification action must be helped by drinking extra water to flush the body of the toxins that are released when the cleansing takes place. Your liver, kidneys, intestines, skin, bladder and lymphatic system will all be working overtime and need as much fluid as possible to dilute the toxins.

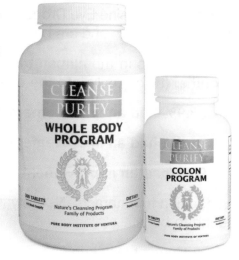

A powerful herbal cleanse may come in two parts. The example shown below is one called "Whole Body & Colon Cleanse Program™."

"Whole Body & Colon Cleanse Program™"

Part 1. **Colon Cleanser** that includes herbs that rid the small intestine and colon of all the putrid matter and mucous that will have built up over the years. The herbs are listed here and you should do your best to obtain one with as many of these herbs as you can find.

> Cascara Sagrada Bark • Rhubarb Root • Calcium Carbonate • Buckthorn Bark • Psyllium Husk • Liquorice Root, Ginger Root • Fennel Seed • Golden Seal Root.

Part 2. **Body Cleanser** that includes herbs to cleanse the whole body including: Liver, Kidneys and Lungs.

> Oregon Grape Root • Mullein Burberry Root • Calcium Carbonate • Black Cohosh Root Dandelion Root • Fenugreek Seed • Prickly Ash Bark • Peppermint Leaf • Ginger Root • Irish Moss • Goldenseal Root • Liquorice Root • Cascara Sagrada Bark Burdock Root • Sarsaparilla Herb • Gentian Root • Yellow Dock Root • Echinacea Root • Safflower Herb • Peach Leaves • Slippery Elm Bark • Chickweed Herb• Yarrow Flower • Capsicum Fruit

The test of a good herbal program is how long you are recommended to cleanse. If it is recommended on the packaging that you need to cleanse for between 1-3 months, then you know you are getting good information, and it should indicate the quality of the products. Even if it includes Milk Thistle in the formulation, you are still recommended to continue with Milk Thistle support for a month or so after you have finished your cleanse. Please note that Milk Thistle should not be used whilst doing the cleanse program

The last stage is to support the liver. The most famous herb for this is Milk Thistle. Doctors and natural health practitioners have used this successfully to help regenerate the liver, when it has been abused and overworked (especially from fats and alcohol).

You will see an example in the data sheets of a liver support program called Revision Formula, and there are many other good herbal formulas available.

As ever, the price will reflect the quality of the product, and you are advised not to buy the cheaper options. Ask for the best.

See the resources page at the end for supplier details.

8. HOMEOPATHY DATA SHEETS

Homeopathy has been used for over 100 years to treat eye diseases as well as many other conditions.

It may be beneficial because:

❖ It works in a good number of cases.
❖ It does not conflict with any of the steps here.
❖ It is relatively easy.
❖ You may get other benefits, especially for emotional issues that may be a concern.
❖ If the practitioner can find your solution it works very quickly (within a few weeks).

The downside is:

❖ There is not a simple list homeopathic remedies that you can buy from the store.
❖ You need to go a qualified practitioner and find what you need specifically.
❖ They will ask you many questions about you to arrive at the best solution for you.

To find a homeopathic practitioner you can:

❖ Ask your doctor to refer you to a Homeopathic doctor.
❖ Search the Internet for the Society of Homeopaths for a listing in your area.

"My eyes are no longer itchy and I have stopped needing to rub them. My eyesight is so much better and I have much more energy."

Mrs. Legge

9. CHELATION AND OZONE DATA SHEETS
Oral Chelation—Serrapeptase
Natural Chelation - Anti-Inflammatory

A Gift from Silkworms

Serrapeptase has had wide clinical use, spanning over twenty-five years throughout Europe and Asia, as a viable alternative to salicylates, ibuprofen and the more potent NSAIDs. Unlike these drugs, Serrapeptase is a naturally occurring, physiologic agent, with no inhibitory effects on prostaglandins, and is devoid of gastrointestinal side effects.

Serrapeptase is a proteolytic enzyme isolated from the microorganism, Serratia E15. This enzyme is naturally present in the silkworm intestine and is processed commercially today through fermentation. This immunologically active enzyme is completely bound to the alpha 2 macroglobulin in biological fluids. Histologic studies reveal powerful anti-inflammatory effects of this naturally occurring enzyme.

Serrapeptase digests nonliving tissue, blood clots, cysts, arterial plaque, and inflammation in all forms.

The late German physician Dr. Hans Nieper used Serrapeptase to treat arterial blockage in his coronary patients. Serrapeptase protects against stroke and is reportedly more effective and quicker than EDTA Chelation treatments in removing arterial plaque. He also reported that Serrapeptase dissolves blood clots and causes varicose veins to shrink or diminish. Dr. Nieper told of a woman scheduled for hand amputation and a man scheduled for bypass surgery who both recovered quickly without surgery after treatment with Serrapeptase.

Dosage:

❖ Treatment of inflammation: 1-3 tablets three times per day on an empty stomach.

❖ Treatment for arterial blockage: 1-3 tablets twice daily.

Uses:

1. Cardiovascular Disease
2. Arthritis
3. Rhumatoid Arthritis
4. Lung Problems
5. Eye Problems
6. Runny Nose and sinusitis problems
7. Sports Injuries
8. Inflammation of any kind

Intravenous Chelation

After more than fifty years of beneficial use on millions of patients in Europe, ozone has been proven to be an effective remedy in the treatment of cancer, arthritis, AIDS, cardiovascular disease, systemic Candidiasis, mononucleosis, hepatitis, herpes, and any other condition of micro-bial contamination. Ozone has also helped improve the nervous system and brain function in senility, multiple sclerosis, Alzheimer's, and Parkinson's disease.

Direct exposure of the blood to ozone can be carried out in a number of ways. The most common and the most popular among German physicians is "Autohemotherapy." A small amount of blood is drawn from the body into a vacuum bottle, after which O3 is infused into the bottle. The bottle is then shaken, and the "ozonated" blood re-infused. Air, which contains nitrogen, never enters the body, so an air embolus cannot occur. In fact, ozone is now carried in ambulances in Germany and administered directly by intravenous injection in patients having just suffered a CVA (stroke). It appears that when ozone is administered within 24 to 48 hours of a stroke, much of the paralysis and other post-stroke complications can be avoided. The use of ozone in spinal cord injury may also prove efficacious in preventing permanent paralysis, by reducing swelling around the spinal cord, but this has yet to be explored.

Laboratory studies have shown that when ozone is introduced into the blood in microgram doses, it is immediately converted into Hydroperoxides, which are free radical scavengers; Glutathione, Catalyse, Super Oxide Dismutase, etc. They have shown remarkable anti-bacterial and anti-fungal effects.

These Hydroperoxides actually seek out and destroy diseased cells and invading organisms and account for ozone's anti-tumor properties.

Infected cells have lower levels of enzyme activity and are less stable. The Hydroperoxides readily react with the cell membrane lipids. Through reaction of ozone with the Phospholipid chains in the cell membrane, Lipoperoxides are introduced into the cell and influence its metabolism; in particular, polyunsaturated fatty acids whose peroxides have a selective Cytotoxic effect and have growth inhibiting effects in human lung, breast, and prostate cancer cells.

Ozone therapy has been in use for many years by thousands of West German doctors who have proven in hundreds of clinical studies that they are able to inactivate AIDS and other viruses through the use of ozone.

There are not very many doctors providing ozone therapy just yet, but if you are suffering from cardiovascular disease, you will benefit with some form of intravenous therapy.

Without this treatment, the recovery of your eyes will be inhibited, and with it, your health will benefit generally.

See the resources page at the end for supplier details.

10. LASER TREATMENTS DATA SHEETS
Laser techniques

These are still not proven and may only apply to a few select sufferers.

It should be considered as a last resort, because it can destroy healthy tissue along with the diseased retina.

If you are one of the lucky few that benefit, and the results are proven to work with no side effects (short or long term), good for you. You must still maintain the health of your eyes, as they will degenerate again and leave you no better off.

It is far better to delay laser treatment until you have given these steps a good chance.

If you are considering laser treatment then here are the questions you MUST ask your physician before YOU decide to proceed with this type of treatment. It is best that you write down the answers to these questions before you make your decision.

1. How many people have been treated nationally with this procedure over the past 5 years? What was the outcome after 1 year? After 5 Years?

2. How many people have you personally treated with this treatment over the past 5 years? What was the outcome after 1 and 5 years?

3. What are the side effects, and what can go wrong? What percentage will suffer these?

4. If I do not have this treatment, will it cause me to be any worse off?

5. If I have this treatment, will it create any lasting damage to healthy tissue?

If you are not prepared to ask these questions, then take along a spokesperson that is happy to ask them for you.

Example Daily Action Sheet

7.00 am on Waking up:

- ❖ With a pint of water, take your Herbal Cleanse.
- ❖ Take Probiotic14 as per label.
- ❖ 15 minutes later, take 4 sprays of Lutein Spray.

Eat Breakfast 30-45 minutes after herbal cleanse. First take digestive enzymes, if you're eating cooked food.

With breakfast:

- ❖ ½ fl.oz. (15ml) of Liquid Vitamins and Minerals.
- ❖ Astaxanthin see label (double dose for first month).
- ❖ Take essential fatty acids oils as per label.

After 1 hour:

- ❖ Drink ½ pint glass of water and a glass every hour until lunch.

Mid-morning:

- ❖ Eat a piece of fruit.
- ❖ 15 minutes later take another 2 sprays of Lutein.

Lunch:

- ❖ 1 hour later drink, ½ pint glass of water and a glass every hour until 30 minutes before evening meal.

Mid-afternoon:

- ❖ Eat another piece of fruit.
- ❖ 15 minutes later take another 2 sprays of Lutein.

½ hour before evening meal:

- ❖ Take Herbal Cleanse with 1 pint of water.

With Evening Meal take:

- ❖ ½ fl.oz (15ml) of Liquid Vitamins and Minerals.
- ❖ Anti-Oxidant Formula as per label (double dose for first month).
- ❖ Take essential fatty acids oils as per label.

After 1 hour:

- ❖ Drink ½ pint of water every hour until 7pm.
- ❖ Take last 4 Lutein sprays.

Late evening snack, 9:30PM:

- ❖ Eat an apple.

Just before bed:

- ❖ Take Probiotic14 as label.

If taking other nutrients such as Taurine please refer to the label.

Remember, chocolate is a reasonably healthy snack.

Research and Studies

Dietary Modification with a Lutein-rich Food Reverses ARMD Vision Loss, According to Optometric Researcher Dr. Stuart Richer

ATLANTA, Feb. 25 /PRNewswire/—Dietary modification with a Lutein-rich food can reverse the damaging effects of age-related macular degeneration (ARMD), the leading cause of blindness in people over age 65 in the United States, according to a report presented today by Stuart Richer, O.D. at the Southern Council of Optometrists 1999 annual meeting. Until this point, research only indicated that diet plays an important role in reducing disease risk.

"Patients demonstrated positive effects in visual function in one or both eyes, with the simple addition of Lutein-rich foods," reported Richer, chief of the Optometry Section, DVA Medical Centre, North Chicago, IL. "This research supports the hypothesis that Lutein is associated with building macular pigment, a key indicator of ARMD risk and pathology."

Richer supplemented the diets of 15 atrophic (dry) ARMD patients with an additional portion of five ounces of sauteed spinach four to seven times per week. Study subjects were given a battery of tests to establish baseline measurements of contrast sensitivity, low-luminance, low-contrast visual acuity, and glare recovery in each eye. Subsequent measurements were made at intervals ranging from two months to 12 months.

Richer observed improvements in visual function in as little as three months. Often striking improvements in vision were detected through follow-up tests, even when the patient did not report subjective vision changes. Partial or complete resolution of metamorphopsia (distorted vision) and scotomas (blind spots) was reported in seven of eight applicable cases.

Dietary treatment of ARMD should receive more attention, due to its simplicity, low cost and potential application in a broad range of ARMD cases, according to Richer. "There is a preoccupation by clinicians and researchers with exudative (wet) ARMD and a continuing commercial and professional interest in higher-technology, expensive treatment approaches," said Richer. "Such therapies are applicable to a small percentage of ARMD patients, and the disease must be detected early for treatment to be effective."

Prevent Blindness America, the nation's leading eye health organization, estimates 13 million people in the U.S. have symptoms of ARMD, and the disease causes visual impairment in 1.2 million. Richer said this is particularly alarming, as the population over the age of 65 is projected to double by the year 2050.

Lutein and Zeaxanthin, related Carotenoids found in leafy green vegetables like spinach and kale, are concentrated in retinal macular pigment, and accumulation is dependent on dietary intake.

Macular pigment may filter blue light that damages photoreceptors and the retinal pigment epithelium. In addition, Carotenoids may limit oxidant stress resulting from metabolism and light, acting as antioxidants.

"There is hope for people who suffer from ARMD, as well as those at risk of the disease. This disease is preventable, and now may even be treatable with the right dietary modifications or intake of Lutein supplements," said Richer.

Improved Nutrition Could Help Prevent Vision Loss

BOSTON—"Vision loss associated with aging may be preventable—even reversible—through improved nutrition," scientists at The Schepens Eye Research Institute said today.

"The traditional thinking is that as age increases, visual sensitivity decreases. But what we are saying is, maybe that's not inevitable," said D. Max Snodderly, Ph.D., head of the laboratory at The Schepens where the research was done. "Improved nutrition could help to retard the loss of visual sensitivity with age. Perhaps the gradual loss of vision in many older people is not an inevitable consequence of the aging process."

In the latest study, Schepens scientists have found that macular pigment in the retina—an accumulation of yellow compounds from fruits and vegetables—may prevent age-related vision loss.

The macula, about the size of a pencil eraser, is at the center of the retina and is responsible for acute vision. Age-related macular degeneration, the leading cause of blindness in people over age 65 in western industrialized nations, occurs when the aging process destroys the macula.

Snodderly, with coauthors Billy Hammond, a former post-doctoral associate now at Arizona State University, Phoenix, and Billy R. Wooten, Professor of Psychology at Brown University, report in Investigative Ophthalmology & Visual Science (Feb. 1998, Vol. 39, No. 2) that macular pigment or dietary factors associated with it appear to protect the retina from loss of sensitivity, when the eye is adapted for light as well as for dark. The National Institutes of Health, the Massachusetts Lions Eye Research Fund, and Kemin Foods funded the research.

Macular pigment is composed of two chemicals, Lutein and Zeaxanthin, that are part of the family of compounds known as Carotenoids. These compounds are contained in plants and protect them from light damage. Particularly high concentrations are contained in dark green and orange plants and fruits, like spinach, broccoli, green beans, corn and peaches, but not carrots. Although carrots are good for Vitamin A deficiency, the retina does not take up beta carotene, which is the main Carotenoid in carrots. "If you eat a lot of fruits and vegetables, you will be getting a lot of Carotenoids," Snodderly said. "This already fits in with public health recommendations for a wide range of health issues—increase intake of vegetables and fruits."

The scientists measured macular pigment and visual sensitivity of 27 healthy older subjects, ages 60 to 84, and compared them with ten younger healthy subjects, ages 24 to 36. Visual sensitivity is how much energy is required to detect photons. Low sensitivity usually associated with aging, means that it is more difficult to see light, and thus, there is some vision loss.

The researchers measured macular pigment density (how much light the pigment absorbs) by flashing blue and green lights in an alternate pattern so the lights appeared to flicker. The blue is absorbed by macular pigment, but not green. The amount of blue light required being equally as effective as the green yields the pigment density.

This technology, which could become an important tool in predicting the risk for macular degeneration, is the subject of a recently filed patent application.

As expected, visual sensitivity declined significantly with age. However, macular pigment was a clear determinant of visual sensitivity: Subjects over age 60 with high macular pigment density had the same visual sensitivity as the younger subjects. Older subjects with low macular pigment density had lower visual sensitivity than the younger subjects.

"The results show that high macular pigment density was associated with the retention of youthful visual sensitivity," the authors write, "which suggested that macular pigment might retard age-related declines in visual function."

Macular pigment density also appears to be correlated with factors that increase the risk of disease, such as age-related macular degeneration: for example, smoking, female gender, and blue irises all are risk factors for the disease, and people with those risk factors also have lower macular pigment density.

Conversely, people with higher macular pigment density are associated with factors that decrease risk, such as high blood concentrations of Carotenoids, high dietary intake of Lutein and Zeaxan-thin, and dark irises.

"Taken together, the evidence suggests that macular pigment may protect against retinal disease by reducing damage that occurs as we age," Snodderly said.

Further, macular pigment density may be useful as a predictor for overall ocular health, the researchers said, because macular pigment density correlates with preservation of clarity of the lens, as well as sensitivity of the retina. Since previous research by others showed that reduced visual sensitivity may predict development of advanced age-related macular degeneration, then, the researchers suggest, increasing macular pigment density might prevent people who are mildly impaired from advancing to the worst stages of the disease.

They write: "It is possible that, by improving protection, retinal or retinal pigment epithelial cells that may be damaged, but still viable, could recover."

Said Snodderly, "It appears that people lose visual sensitivity before the worst stages of disease. But with the right nutritional program, you might prevent the low macular pigment group from getting worse, and in the best cases even recover some of the lost function."

The research also has resulted in a way to tailor dietary recommendations to an individual, the scientists said.

"Our studies have suggested that individuals differ in their ability to absorb nutrients from food into their tissues," Hammond said. "Thus, some individuals can have relatively high intake of fruits and vegetables and high nutrient blood levels but actually low levels of retinal nutrients. The ability to easily measure macular pigment in vivo may allow us to identify such individuals and determine whether they are at special risk for disease. In the future we may be able to use such technology to tailor our dietary recommendations based on individual responses rather than relying on averaged effects."

The three treatment groups (10 mg Lutein, 10 mg Lutein plus antioxidants and placebo) were matched for: age, years diagnosed with AMD, smoking/cardiovascular history, iris color, lens opacif(cation, and nutritional status/physical activity level.

Average eye MPOD, as measured by heterochromic flicker photometry, increased on average by 0.09 log units (repeated factors ANOVA; $p<0.05$), or 50 % in both the Lutein and Lutein plus antioxidant treatment groups by 12 months. There was statistically significant concurrent improvement in some measures of visual function, including GR, CSF, and distance/near visual acuity in both treatment groups. Crossover, double crossover, and video-documentation of patient symptoms pre- and post-treatment were consistent with objective data. Inclusion of multiple nutrients (besides Lutein) appears to provide an added improvement to CSF.

Summary of the main outcome of the LAST relatively to the placebo group.

- ❖ Lutein—Macular Pigment Optical Density (MPOD)—50% increase by 12 months

- ❖ Lutein plus an Antioxidant—Macular Pigment Optical Density (MPOD)—50% increase by 12 months

Conclusions:

Reversibility of ARMD symptoms has important biophysical, physiological, and clinical implications. This population prospective clinical trial agrees with previous studies suggesting ARMD to be a nutrition-responsive disorder. The authors believe that low technology visual evaluation protocols, combined with Lutein-based nutritional intervention recommendations, may improve the eye health of older patients with the dry form of ARMD.

Lutein, essential for eyesight and other conditions

(from a recent publication - unknown author)

Without your vision, you would not be reading this sentence. Even so, we often take our eyesight for granted, paying less attention to our eyes than to our thoughts. But the truth is that many people are at risk of at least partial loss of eyesight and other vision problems.

The human eye is 1/6th the size of the heart, yet uses 60 times as much oxygen, and requires more nutrition to maintain healthy tissue and function than any other organ in the body.

There are four main causes of vision impairment or disability, they are: Glaucoma, Diabetic Retin-opathy, Cataracts, and Macular Degeneration.

As we age, changes take place in our eyes. Lifelong exposure to light can lead to a decrease in the number of photoreceptors (light sensitive nerves) in the eye. Sunlight and fluorescent light can produce free radicals which break down, or oxidize, the fatty substances that make up the outer segments or "photoreceptors." This process eventually damages the retina, the paper-thin tissue lining the back of the eyeball.

Another age-related problem is the growth of tiny blood vessels over the central area of the retina, where visual perception is most acute. These changes are related to aging, as well as unprotected exposure to sunlight and continual eye muscle strain—but they are not inevitable.

The good news is, it's now possible to protect the eyes with nutrition. "It's been estimated that with proper antioxidant defense, the human eye is capable of staying healthy all through your life," reports the New Science Nutrition Magazine.

Of specific importance for reducing the risk, and alleviating the problems of Cataracts and Macular Degeneration, are three members of the Carotenoid family:

Lutein

One of the newest discoveries in nutritional research is the role of the Carotenoid Lutein. Carotenoids are botanical pigments that give certain plants their distinctive red, orange, and yellow colors. Beyond their broad-spectrum antioxidant activity, Carotenoids have an affinity for specific organs in the body. In the case of Lutein (the pigment that gives a sunny yellow color to corn and marigolds), that organ is the eye.

Nature, in its wisdom, has concentrated Lutein in the macular region of the retina and the lens, where it is most needed to protect against photo-oxidation (free radical damage). This is because the process of vision involves light being focused through the lens onto the retina. The macula or centre of the retina receives the most light. Its millions of cells, which provide the sharp vision needed to see clearly, are bombarded with light on a daily basis.

Light is an oxidant; when it strikes the fatty acid of the macular region, damage can occur. Lutein, a potent antioxidant, can help maintain the integrity of the macular tissue where it is concentrated, and also protect the blood vessels that supply the macular region.

It is recommended Lutein be taken with food with a low fat content for best absorption. This does not apply if taking the sublingual Lutein spray, which ensures perfect absorption.

Zeaxanthin

This is found in the same foods as Lutein, and has most of the same beneficial effects. Lutein can also convert into Zeaxanthin.

Beta Carotene

A powerful antioxidant that also has a beneficial effect on the retina.

Severe deficiency can cause visual problems, including double vision, impaired vision, and over time, blindness.

Lutein and Zeaxanthin are the only Carotenoids and the most dominant pigments in the macular region of the retina and the lens. Their antioxidant properties help maintain the integrity of the blood vessels that supply the macular region of the retina, providing protection from photo-oxidation, the result of light striking the fatty acids in the retina. Lutein is particularly active in absorbing the blue part of the light spectrum, which can be the most damaging to our eyes.

How Lutein And Zeaxanthin Work

In the eye, light passes through the lens and hits the retina located at the back of the eye. The retina transforms these light images into electrical impulses, which are transmitted to the brain by the optic nerve.

In the center of the retina is a small, oval shaped area called the macula, which governs detail in our vision. Within the macula is the macular pigment, which filters out harmful "blue light" that generates damaging free radicals in the eye. The macular pigment is made up primarily of Lutein and Zeaxanthin, suggesting that these nutrients are crucial to good eye health.

Essentially, Lutein and Zeaxanthin contribute to the density of macular pigment. The denser the pigment, the more protection there is.

Proof Of The Study

❖ A study at the Department of Chemistry, Florida International University, was carried out to determine the effects of dietary supplementation with Lutein on macular pigment density. Two groups consumed the equivalent of 30mg of Lutein per day for a period of 140 days. Twenty to forty days after the subjects commenced taking the Lutein supplement, their macular pigment density began to increase. At the end of the test period, the subjects experienced a 30-40% reduction in blue light reaching the photoreceptors, Bruch's membrane and the retinal pigment epithelium - the vulnerable tissues affected by Age-Related Macular Degeneration (ARMD).

"Over 25 epidemiological studies examining dietary intake of Carotenoids found that Lutein and Zeaxanthin are inversely associated with age-related macular degeneration," said Andrew Shao, technical services manager for vitamins and dietary supplements at Kemin Foods.

❖ A study using Lutein supplements resulted in a 15% increase in macular pigment levels after 72 days. In another study, people who consumed the equivalent of 6 mg of Lutein per day were 40% less likely to experience macular problems.

❖ Another study, using sets of identical twins, demonstrated that macular Lutein concentrations were related to dietary Lutei.

❖ In a Multi-Centre Eye Disease Case-Control Study in the United States of 356 patients with macular degeneration and 520 controls, aged 55 to 80 years old, those in the highest quintile of Carotenoid intake had a 43% lower risk of Macular Degeneration compared to individuals in the lowest quintile. Zeaxanthin and Lutein were the Carotenoids most strongly associated with decreased risk. Those who had the highest intake of Lutein and Zeaxanthin had a 57% lower risk of Macular Degeneration.

❖ In a study of the correlation between antioxidant status and senile cataracts in 112 subjects aged 40 to 70 years old in the USA, high plasma levels of at least two of the three antioxidant vitamins, E, C and Carotenoids, were associated with a significantly reduced risk of cataract development, compared to low levels of at least one of these vitamins. Subjects with high plasma antioxidant status had an 80% decrease in cataract risk.

❖ Another study examined 493 participants from the Nurses Health Study who had undergone cataract extraction between 1984 and 1986. The researchers found that women who had a higher total Carotenoid intake had a lower risk of developing cataracts than those with the lowest intake of Carotenoids. Furthermore, cataract risk was 47% to 65% lower in women who ate spinach and other greens five or more times per week.

❖ In a 1994 Harvard Study, people who consumed fruits and vegetables containing Lutein had a 43% reduction in the risk of Macular Degeneration.

❖ In November 2000, the Journal of Investigative Ophthalmology and Visual Science reported that researchers gave eight male subjects 10mg of Lutein for 12 weeks. All the subjects showed a substantial increase in plasma Lutein concentration.

Proprietary research by Sloan, Trends & Solitons found the number one health concern for consumers is eyesight. Age-related Macular Degeneration is the leading cause of acquired blindness in the USA, afflicting 1.4 million Americans alone. In addition, 6.4 million people suffer from cataracts, the leading cause of vision impairment. It is estimated that by 2030, over 40% of the UK population will be 45 and older, and will be concerned about ARMD.

The British Medical Journal in1992 reported the results of an 8-year study on 50,000 women and showed those who regularly had a diet containing Lutein and Zeaxanthin had a much lower level of cataract formation.

Lutein Protects More Than The Eyes

As well as protecting your eyes, Lutein can provide protection from heart disease and cancer. Lutein, is in fact, one of the top five nutritional products to help protect you from heart disease, cancer, and eye disease, particularly ARMD.

ARMD and Heart Diseases

Just 6 mg of Lutein daily could reduce the incidence of Macular Degeneration by as much as 43%. In the vascular system, Lutein is found in HDL, or "good" cholesterol, and may prevent LDL or "bad" cholesterol from accelerating, which sets the cascade for heart disease.

Cancers

Studies have shown Lutein is associated with a reduction in lung and cervical cancers. While most of the research on Lutein looks at its benefits for the eyes and heart, researchers have also studied its relationship to cancer. University of Michigan researchers, for example, found that Lutein was the most predominant Carotenoid in the cervix of the healthy women they studied.

Lutein, also essential to combat:

- ❖ Macular Degeneration
- ❖ Cataracts
- ❖ Breast Cancer
- ❖ LDL Cholesterol
- ❖ Diabetic Retinopathy
- ❖ Lung Cancer
- ❖ Glaucoma
- ❖ Heart Disease
- ❖ Colon Cancer
- ❖ Premature Ageing

Lutein, they discovered, is rapidly metabolized in the cervix of women. Their work led them to conclude that a higher intake of Lutein offers protection from cervical cancer. Like the macula and lens of the eye, a woman's cervix undergoes a lot of oxidative stress, which changes not only vital cells but also DNA itself! This conclusion supports earlier studies showing a decreased prevalence of cervical cancer among women who consumed diets high in fruits and vegetables.

Other studies, of women with breast cancer, show a strong relationship between Carotenoid intake and an improved prognosis. Once again, researchers believe a high intake of yellow and green vegetables containing Lutein was responsible.

Lutein's protective effect on cancer doesn't stop with cervical and breast cancer. There is impressive data to show that lung cancer rates are also lower among those who consume more Lutein. For example, people in the Fijian Islands who eat an average of 18-23 mg of Lutein per day have considerably fewer cases of lung cancer than those on other South Pacific Islands, where the inhabitants consume much less Lutein, and the rate of smoking is the same.

RECENT LUTEIN RESEARCH 1992-1997

1992—An association between eating foods high in Carotenoids, a high level of Carotenoids in the blood and a lower incidence of macular degeneration is established. (9) The Nurse's Health Study reported a high dietary intake of spinach and other greens with high levels of the specific Carotenoids Lutein and Zeaxanthin led to a 27-39% reduced risk of cataract formation. (10)

1993— Data suggested a reduced risk of neovascular AMD in persons with higher levels of serum Carotenoids. (11)

1994— Dr. Seddon found that eating foods high in Lutein led to a reduced risk for macular degeneration. (2)

1995— Dr. Yeum reported Lutein and Zeaxanthin as the only two Carotenoid antioxidants found in the lens and retina. (1)

1997— Studies were published showing a 30% reduced macular pigment density with AMD and cataracts. A correlation was found between reduced macular pigment density and increased lens density (cataracts) in seniors. (12)(13) With dietary and/or supplemental Lutein, macular pigment density can be increased. (14)

JOURNAL REFERENCES

1. KJ Yeum et al. 1995 Investigative Ophthalmology & Visual Science 36:2756-61.

2. JM Seddon et al. 1994 Journal of the American Medical Association 272:1420.

3. F Khachik et al. 1995 Journal of Cellular Biochemistry 22:236-46.

4. LH Zhang et al. 1991 Carcinogenesis 12:2109-14.

5. DM Snodderly 1995 American Journal of Clinical Nutrition 62S:1448S-61S.

6. Chopra et al. 1994 Proc Nutritional Society 53:18A.

7. Goulient et al. 1997 Arterioscleroses Thrombosis Vascular Biology 17:4:786-96.

8. LE Marchand et al. 1995 International Journal of Cancer 63:18-23.

9. Eye Disease Control Study Group 1992 Archives of Ophthalmology 110:1701-8.

10. Hankinson et al. 1992 British Medical Journal 305:335-9.

11. Eye Disease Control Study Group 1993 Archives of Ophthalmology 111:104-9.

12. JT Landrum et al. 1997 Advances in Pharmacology 38:537-56.11

13. BR Hammond, Jr. et al. 1997 Optometry and Vision Science 74:7:499-504.

14. BR Hammond, Jr. et al.1997 Investigative Ophthalmology & Visual Science 38:1795-1801.

MACULAR DEGENERATION STUDIES

1. A preliminary study showed those consuming Lutein from either spinach or supplements demonstrated improvement of some of the early vision loss from "dry" macular degeneration. Richer, J. Amer Optom Assoc; Jan 1999.

2. Consuming 6 mg of the Caroteinoid Lutein (with its co-nutrient Zeaxanthin) daily for five months was shown to significantly increase macular pigment density, which protects from harmful blue wavelength light believed to be most responsible for macular degeneration. Landrum, et al. Exp Eye Res 1997 Jul;65(1):57-62

3. High macular pigment density was associated with the retention of youthful visual sensitivity, which suggested that increasing macular pigment might retard age-related declines in visual function. Hammond, et al. Invest Ophthalmol Vis Sci 1997 Aug; 38(9): 1795-801.

4. Persons who had the lowest serum levels of Lycopene, the most abundant Carotenoid in the serum, were twice as likely to have macular degeneration when compared to those with the highest levels. Mares-Perlman, et al. Arch Ophthalmol 1995 Dec;113(12):1518-23

5. Those consuming Lutein rich foods (spinach and collard greens) five days per week were 8 times less likely to develop macular degeneration as those consuming them once per month. Seddon, et al. JAMA 1994 Nov 9;272(18):1413-20

6. The ARMD population manifested decreased intake of vitamin E, magnesium, zinc, vitamin B6 and folic acid. Patients with advanced ARMD taking antioxidants twice daily maintained vision in their better functioning eyes significantly better than those taking a placebo. Richer, J Am Optom Assoc 1996 Jan;67(1):12-29-J Am Optom Assoc 1996 Jan;67(1):30-49

7. Smokers with early macular degeneration who consumed the lowest amounts of Carotenoids were nearly six times as likely to develop advanced macular degeneration than those consuming the highest amounts. Seddon, et al. J. Amer Med Assoc; 1994.

8. In a clinical trial 60% of subjects with ARMD or diabetic macular oedema who received 500 mg of vitamin C, 400 IU of vitamin E, 15,000 IU of beta-carotene and selenium showed either improvement or no further progression of their disease. So Med J, 1987.

9. The evidence suggests that Carotenoids and antioxidant vitamins may help to retard some of the destructive processes in the retina and the retinal pigment epithelium that are responsible for age-related degeneration of the macula. Am J Clin Nutr 1995 Dec;62(6 Suppl):1448S-1461S

10. The minerals copper and zinc are required to synthesize superoxide dismutase and other enzymes in the retina which scavenge free radicals, preventing the oxidative damage which plays a role in the development of drusen, an early sign of Age-Related Macular Degeneration. Olin, et al: Proc Soc Exp Biol Med 1995 Apr;208(4):370-7

11. Glutathione and its related enzyme precursor amino acids (N-Acetyl-Cysteine, L-Glycine, and glutamine and selenium) are protective against damage to human retinal pigment epithelium cells. Sternberg, Davidson, Jones, et al. Invest Ophthalmol Vis Sci 1993 Dec;34(13):3661-8

12. Quercetin protected bovine retinas in vitro from induced lipid peroxidation, especially when combined with vitamin E, suggesting a potential protective effect in age-related macular degeneration. Ophthalmic Res 1996;28(3):184-92.

13. Deficiency of Taurine, an amino acid, has been shown to lead to retinal degeneration and supplementing it has been used with some success to prevent, treat and stabilise retinal changes. Altern Med Rev 1998 Apr;3(2):128-36.-Oftalmol Zh 1989;(8):463-5- Brain Res Brain Res Rev 1991 May-Aug;16(2):151-69- J Neurosci Res 1987;18(4):602-14

14. After 18 months, subjects with macular degeneration who took antioxidants on a consistent basis were two and a half times more likely to improve on visual acuity testing, and four times less likely to deteriorate in their worst eye, compared to those who took them less consistently. Olson, et al. J. Cat Refr Surg, Mar 1991.

15. Patients with confluent soft drusen, or "pre-wet" ARMD, were found to have evidence of vitamin B6 deficiency. B. Lane, Ann Mtg Amer Coll of Nutrition, 1991.

16. General measures for prevention and remediation of macular degeneration would include a combination of supplementation with trace elements, antioxidants and other vitamins, ...increasing physical fitness, improving nutrition (e.g. avoiding hydrogenated oils), abstaining from smoking, and protection from excessive light exposure. Eur J Med Res 1997 Oct 30;2(10):445-54

17. There is an association between both low serum selenium levels and current smoking status and the development of age-related macular degeneration. Doc Ophthalmol 1992;81(4):387-400- Mayer, et al. Acta Ophthalmol Scand 1998 Feb;76(1):62-7-

18. There was an inverse relationship between dietary pro-vitamin A Carotenoid and vitamin E consumption and the incidence of large macular drusen, as well as between zinc levels and the incidence of retinal pigment abnormalities. Am J Epidemiol 1998 Jul 15;148(2):204-14

19. The evidence suggests that Carotenoids and antioxidant vitamins may help to retard some of the destructive processes in the retina and the retinal pigment epithelium that lead to age-related degeneration of the macula. Snodderly, Am J Clin Nutr 1995;62(6 suppl):1448S-61S

20. Subnormal zinc and/or vitamin E serum levels may be associated with as much as an 82% increased risk of advanced age-related macular degeneration.-Vitamin C and Lipoic acid help to recycle vitamin E in the retinal tissues. Ishihara, et al.-Nippon Ganka Gakkai Zasshi 1997-Mar;101(3):248-51. Delcourt C. et al. Arch Ophthalmol 1999 Oct;117(10):1384-90-Stoyanovsky DA, et al. Curr Eye Res 1995 Mar;14(3):181-9

22. In a study of adults over 60 there was found to be a significant link between risk of macular degeneration and low blood levels of vitamin E as well as increased sun exposure. Belda, et al Mech Ageing Dev 1999 Mar 1;107(2):159-64

23. A statistically significant improvement in visual acuity was observed after treatment with Ginkgo Biloba extract in a double blind, placebo controlled study of macular degeneration patients. Lebuisson DA, et al.-Presse Med 1986 Sep 25;15(31):1556-8

24. Those consuming fish more than once per week were only half as likely to develop macular degeneration than those consuming it less than once per month. Those consuming the highest amount of cholesterol in their diet were 2.7 times more likely to develop advanced macular degeneration. Smith, et al. Arch Ophthalmol 2000 Mar;118(3):401-4

25. Dietary enzymes increase Glutathione synthesis that can prevent free radical-induced apoptosis (cell suicide) and may help prevent or treat AMD. Progress in Retinal and Eye Research, 2000, Vol. 19, Iss.2 pp 205-221 (No abstract available)

GLAUCOMA STUDIES

1. In a study of open angle glaucoma patients who received 150mg of Alpha Lipoic Acid each day, 45-47% of the eyes had enhancement of colour visual fields and visual sensitivity when compared to controls using only topical medical therapy. More advanced cases had an even better response compared to their controls. Filina, et al., Vestn Oftalmol 1995 Oct-Dec;111(4):6-8

2. Pre-treatment with Alpha Lipoic acid has been found to reduce neuronal damage from excitotoxic damage from cyanide, glutamate and iron ions, demonstrating a strong neuroprotective effect for this substance in nerve tissue. It may be useful in treating

glaucoma.-(Ed. Note: Recent evidence points to the importance of neuroprotection against glutamate in glaucoma patients, with many medications now heavily promoting this property!) J Cereb Blood Flow Metab 1995 Jul;15(4):624-30-Altern Med Rev 1998 Aug;3(4):308-11 (Other ALA/Neuroprotective Studies)

3. The eyes of open angle glaucoma patients were found to have significantly lower vitamin C levels, as well as higher levels of lipic peroxidation by-products compared to normals. Aleksidze, et al. Oftalmol Zh 1989;(2):114-6-

4. Patients suffering from open angle glaucoma and normal-tension glaucoma that were given magnesium twice daily showed improvement of the visual field and reduced peripheral vasospasms (which can cause glaucoma, stroke and heart attack) after four weeks of treatment. Gaspar, et al; Ophthalmologica 1995;209(1):11-3

5. Glaucoma patients treated with vitamin B12 for over 5 years demonstrated better visual acuity and better overall control of their disease. Glacome, 1992; Nippon Ganka Kiyo. 1965 Mar.; Oftalmol Zh. 1965; 20(6); Klin Oczna 1974 Nov;44(11):1183-7

6. Besides beta-carotene, other Carotenoids found in dark green leafy vegetables appear to be much more essential to the health of the eye. Several studies have shown that Lutein and Zeaxanthin supplements may slow vision loss in glaucoma, and in some cases improve eyesight. Science News, Volume 146.

7. Anthocyanosides, compounds found in the herb bilberry, were shown to markedly improve vascular resistance of the capillary wall in the ciliary body of the eye (the source of excess fluid production). Boll. Ocul. 65 789-95, 1986

8. Chronic open angle glaucoma patients had a statistically significant lower thiamine blood level than controls along with-poor absorption of that nutrient. Asregadoo, Ann Ophthalmol 1979 Jul;11(7):1095-1100

9. Lipoic acid may be useful in the treatment of glaucoma and may help prevent ischemic optic nerve damage. Altern Med Rev 1998 Aug;3(4):308-11

10. The scientific literature supports recommending Lipoic acid in complex with vitamins B1, B2, B5, B6 (pyridoxal phosphate), and vitamin C to glaucoma patients. Filina, AA & Sporova, NA. Vestn Oftalmol 1991 May-Jun;107(3):19-21

11. Vascular obstruction and hindrance of the blood flow and impaired nutrition of neuronal tissue might be the primary causes of glaucoma. Sonnsjo & Krakau, Acta Ophthalmol (Copenh) 1993 Aug;71(4):433-44

12. Ginkgo Biloba is a potentially important agent in the treatment of glaucoma.-It improves central and peripheral blood flow, reduces vasospasm, reduces serum viscosity, has antioxidant activity, platelet activating factor inhibitory activity, and inhibits apoptosis and excitotoxicity - all factors in preventing glaucoma vision loss. (Ed. Note: magnesium also has been shown to decrease peripheral vasospasms, improving blood flow and is neuroprotective, as well.) Ritch R. Med Hypotheses 2000 Feb;54(2):221-35

13. The fatty acid DHA (abundant in fish oil), along with B Complex and vitamin E were shown to be helpful in preventing or delaying vision loss associated with glaucoma. Cellini M, et al., Acta Ophthalmol Scand Suppl 1998;(227):41

14. Ginkgo Biloba extract (40mg, three times daily), increased diastolic blood flow by 23% in the ophthalmic artery in glaucoma patients and may be helpful in protecting the optic nerve from further damage and subsequent visual field loss. Chung HS, et al. J Ocul Pharmacol Ther 1999 Jun;15(3):233-40-(NB: Ginkgo must be used with caution by those taking Coumadin, as it may increase its effect—possibly eliminating the need for it?)

15. Besides Alpha Lipoic Acid, other nutrients that are neuroprotective include vitamin E, ginkgo Biloba, pycnogenol (from grape seed extract or pine bark), and flavonoids. Kobayashi MS, et al. Free Radic Res 2000 Feb;32(2):115-24

DIABETIC EYE STUDIES

1. Alpha Lipoic Acid can significantly reduce diabetic cataract formation, as well as neuropathy, and would seem to be an ideal neuroprotective substance in the treatment of all oxidative brain and neural disorders involving free radical processes. Packer, L., Ann N Y Acad Sci 1994 Nov 17;738:257-64-Packer, L. Free Radic Biol Med 1997;22(1-2):359-78-

2. Vitamin E significantly improved glucose tolerance in non-insulin dependent diabetics, which should very likely result in fewer diabetic complications. Paolisso, G, et al. Am J Clin Nutr 1993; 57:650-56.

3. Diabetic patients with high serum magnesium levels were less likely to develop severe diabetic retinopathy compared to those with low levels. Diabetes 1978 Nov;27(11):1075-7.

4. Chromium, high-dose vitamin E, magnesium, soluble fibre, and possibly Taurine appear likely to lessen risk for macrovascular disease (retinopathy) in diabetics. McCarty, Med Hypotheses 1997 Aug;49(2):143-52.

5. Bioflavonoids, including those from bilberry extract, were found to normalise blood vessels' permeability in diabetic patients, probably reducing the risk of diabetic retinopathy. Valenci, et al. Diabet Med 1996 Oct;13(10):882-8.-Detre, et al. Clin Physiol Biochem 1986;4(2):143-9

6. Seven of fifteen patients with Type I diabetic retinopathy who were given vitamin B12 along with their daily insulin injections were found to have complete regression of retinal signs after 12 months. Kornerup T, Strom L. Acta Paediatr 1958.

7. 79% of 37 patients with visible diabetic retinal abnormalities improved after taking 160 mg of bilberry extract twice daily, compared to 0% of the placebo control group, and 86% of those with abnormalities of angiography findings showed moderate to considerable improvement.-(These improvements were noted within one month.) Perossini, et al.-Ann Ottalmol Clin Ocul 1987.

8. 73% of type I and II diabetics who took chromium supplements reduced their requirement for insulin or oral hypoglycaemic agents.-Taking chromium and niacin together reduced fasting blood sugar levels and improved glucose tolerance. J Trace Elem Exp Med 1995: 8:183-90;-Urberg M, Zemel MB, Metabolism 1987; 36:896-99.

9. Low magnesium levels might increase the risk of ischemic heart disease and severe retinopathy in diabetics, while chromium increases insulin sensitivity and raises the 'good' HDL cholesterol. Tuvemo, T. Pediatrician 1983-85;12(4):213-9

10. Low serum Carotenoid levels were found to be directly related to an increased risk for developing insulin resistance and diabetes. Ford, et al. Am J Epidemiol 1999 Jan 15;149(2):168-76

11. Both Panax and American ginseng was shown to normalise glucose tolerance tests, and reduced blood sugar spikes in Type II diabetics after consumption of a sugar solution. Vuksan V, et al., Arch Intern Med 2000 Apr 10;160(7):1009-13

12. In one study all 38 patients with insulin-dependent diabetes were required to lower their insulin dose to avoid hypoglycaemia after taking-200mg of Gymnema Sylvestre extract twice daily. Shanmugasundaram ER, et al. J Ethnopharmacol 1990 Oct;30(3):281-94

CATARACT STUDIES

1. Subjects taking vitamin C supplements for more than 10 years had a 45-77% lower risk of early lens opacities (cataracts) and 83% lower risk of moderate lens opacities. The higher the serum levels, the lower the risk of cataracts. Jacques, et al. The American Journal of Clinical Nutrition, Oct. 1997. S.E. Hankinson, et al. 1992. BMJ: 305: 335-339.-Simon JA, Hudes ES J Clin Epidemiol 1999 Dec;52(12):1207-11

2. Vitamin E, vitamin C, alpha-Lipoic acid, and Taurine appear to offer protection against lens damage caused by low-level radiation. Bantseev, et al. Biochem Mol Biol Int 1997 Sep;42(6):1189-97.

3. Dietary Lutein and cryptoxanthin were associated with 70% lower risk of nuclear cataracts in those under age 65. Lyle, et al. Am J Clin Nutr 1999 Feb;69(2):272-7.

4. Dietary intake of protein, vitamins A, C, E, and carotene, niacin, riboflavin, and thiamine significantly decreased the risk of all cataract types.-(Combining a variety of antioxidant nutrients produced the greatest effect.) Cumming RG, et al. Ophthalmology 2000 Mar;107(3):450-6-Leske, et al. Arch Ophthalmol 1991 Feb;109(2):244-51.

5. Vitamin E taken with bilberry extract stopped the progression of senile cortical cataracts in 97% of the eyes of human subjects. Ann Ottalmol Clin Ocul, 1989.

6. Low blood levels of vitamin E were associated with approximately twice the risk of both cortical and nuclear cataracts, compared to median or high levels. Vitale, et al. Epidemiology 1993 May;4(3):195-203-

7. Smokers were 2.6 times as likely to develop posterior sub capsular cataracts than non-smokers. Hankinson, et al. JAMA 1992 Aug 26;268(8):994-8

8. Patients with senile cataracts were found to have significantly lower blood and intraocular levels of the mineral selenium than controls. Karakucuk S, et al.-Acta Ophthalmol Scand 1995 Aug;73(4):329-32

9. Alpha Lipoic acid can help prevent cataract formation as well as nerve degeneration and radiation injury. Packer, et al. Free Radic Biol Med 1995 Aug;19(2):227-50

RETINITIS PIGMENTOSA STUDIES

1. Patients with retinitis pigmentosa appear to have faulty cellular uptake of the amino acid Taurine.-Disturbed utilisation of vitamin A also appears to play a part in retinitis pigmentosa,

and a subgroup of patients benefit from supplementation of this vitamin. Head KA, Altern Med Rev 1999 Oct;4(5):342-59

1. The essential fatty acids alpha-Linolenic acid and DHA may be required for those with retinitis pigmentosa to support normal functional development of the retina. Uauy R, et al. Lipids 1996 Mar;31 Suppl:S167-76-

1. A diet high in polyunsaturated fats (e.g. corn oil), and low in vitamin E, selenium, sulphur-containing amino acids (e.g. Taurine, methionine),-and chromium were related to a build up of pigment that mimics one type of retinitis pigmentosa. Katz, et al. Invest Ophthalmol Vis Sci 1978

1. Lutein supplementation in high doses improved both visual acuities and visual fields after 2-4 weeks of treatment in 16 subjects, and was especially effective in blue-eyed individuals. Dagnelie G., et al-Optometry 2000 Mar;71(3):147-64

Alpha Lipoic Acid REFERENCES

1. Berkson, B., The Alpha Lipoic Acid Breakthrough, Prima Publishing, Rocklin, CA, 1998.

2. Biewenga, G., Haenen G., Bast, A., "The pharmacology of the antioxidant Lipoic acid", Gen. Pharmacol. 1997 Sept; 29(3): 315-31

3. Jacob, S., et al. "Enhancement of glucose disposal in patients with type 2 diabetes by Alpha-Lipoic acid". Arzn.-Forsch, 1995;45:872-4.

4. Ziegler D., Gries, F., "Alpha-Lipoic Acid in the treatment of diabetic peripheral and cardiac autonomic neuropathy", Diabetes, 1997 Sept46 Supp12562.6.

5. Meletis, C., "Basic Nutrient Support for Proper Immune Function". Alternative & Complementary Therapies, Feb. 1999, p.44.

6. Konrad, T., et al "Alpha Lipoic Acid treatment decreases serum lactate and pyruvate concentrations and improves glucose effectiveness in lean and obese patients with type 2 diabetes", Diabetes Care. 1999 Feb; 22(2): 280-7.

7. Whiteman, M., et al. "Protection against peroxynitrite-dependent tyrosine nitration and al-anti-proteinase inactivation by oxidised and reduced lipoic acid", FEBS Letters, 1996; 379:74-6.

8. Wickramasinghe, S., Hasan, R, "In Vitro Effects of Vitamin C, Thioctic Acid and Dihydrolipoic Acid on the Cytotoxicity of Post-Ethanol Serum", Biochemical Pharmacology, 1992; 43(3): 407-11.

9. Maitra, I, et al "Alpha-Lipoic acid prevents buthionine sulfoximine — Induced cataract formation in newborn Rats", Free Radical Biology & Medicine, 1995-18:823-829.

10. Bustamante, J., et al "Antioxidant inhibition of thymocyte apoptosis by Dihydrolipoic acid", Free Radical Biol. & Med, 1995; 19:339-47.

11. Barbiroli, B., et al. "Lipoic (thioctic acid) increases brain energy available and skeletal muscle performance as shown in vivo 31:-MRS in a patient with mitochondrial cytopathy", J. Neurol., 1995;242:472-7.

12. Schonhit, K, et al. "Effect of Alpha-Lipoic Acid and Dihydrolipoic acid on ischemia/

reperfuslon injury of the heart and heart mitochondria", Biochimica et Biophysics Acta., 1995; 1271:335-42.

13. Greenamyre, J., et al. "The endogenous cofactors, thioctic acid and Dihydrolipoic acid, are neuroprotective against NMDA and malonlc acid Lesions of striatum", Neuroscience Letters, 1994; 171:17-20

14. Mitsui, Y, et al "Alpha-Lipoic acid provides neuroprotection from ischemla-reperfusion injury of peripheral nerve", J. Neuro. Sci., Feb. 1; 163(1): 11-6.

15. Stol S., et al. "The potent free radical scavenger Alpha Lipoic Acid improves memory in aged mice: putative relationship to NMDA receptor deficits", Pharmacol, Biochem.& Behavior, 1993: 46:799.805.

DOCTORS REPORTS

Dr Ed Kondrot, a leading ophthalmic surgeon in the USA, believes Lutein and micro-current stimulation can actually reverse the damage in people who have lost most of their sight. He says, "We have a number of examples of patients who were forced to give up driving because of their Macular Degeneration, but who can now drive again".

Grace Halloran PhD, a research scientist, who had lost her sight as a result of Retinitis Pigmentosa (a genetic condition), regained her vision after taking Lutein supplementation and using micro-current stimulation. She says, "It is not perfect—a little foggy—but I can get around now, whereas before I could not see a thing."

From the Web Site of Damon P. Miller II, M.D., N.D.—Results of the first 120 people he treated with Microcurrent Stimulation:

> "We have been treating people with retinal disease in this office for two years now, and have just analyzed the results from the first 120 patients that we treated. The results have been quite gratifying. One surprise that we find in analyzing the data is how well the people with the wet form of aged-related macular degeneration have responded."

Results

> "Of all 120 patients treated, 83% (101/120) showed improvement of greater than, or equal to, two lines of visual acuity in one or both eyes. If we include those who had at least one line of improvement in visual acuity, then 93% showed improvement.

> "There were 11 patients (11 of 120) with Stargardt's Disease who were treated, and, of these, all 11 or 100% showed an improvement of greater than, or equal to, two lines of visual improvement in one or both eyes.

> "There was one patient (1 of 120) who had the diagnosis of X-linked Retinoschisis, who also showed two lines of improvement on visual acuity testing in both eyes.

> "If we take the 109 patients with aged-related macular degeneration (ARMD), and break them down by diagnosis type into exudative (wet) and non-exudative (dry), we find that of the patients with wet ARMD, 88% (43/49) showed an improvement of two lines or greater on visual acuity testing. Of those with dry ARMD, 77% (46/60) showed improvement of two lines or more on visual acuity testing."

CARNOSINE STUDY

Moscow Helmholtz Research Institute of Eye Diseases, Russian Federation.

The naturally occurring compound N alpha-acetylcarnosine (NAC) is proposed as the prodrug of L-carnosine (C) resistant to enzymatic hydrolysis by human serum carnosinase. Rabbit eyes were treated with 1% NAC, C, or placebo and extracts of the aqueous humor from the anterior eye chamber were analyzed for imidazole content by reverse phase analytical high performance liquid chromatography (HPLC), thin-layer (TLC) and ion-exchange chromatographic techniques. The topical administration of pure C to the rabbit eye did not lead to accumulation of this compound in the aqueous humor over 30 min in concentration exceeding that in the placebo-treated matched eye. MAC showed dose-dependent hydrolysis in its passage from the cornea to the aqueous humor, releasing C after 15. 30 min of ocular administration of prodrug in a series of therapeutical modalities: instillation < or = subconjunctival injection < or = ultrasound induced phoresis. Different treatment techniques showed excellent toleration of 1% MAC by the eye.

Once in the aqueous humor, C might act as an antioxidant and enter the lens tissue when present at effective concentrations (5-15 mmol/l). The advantage of the ophthalmic prodrug MAC and its bioactivated principle C as universal antioxidants relates to their ability to give efficient protection against oxidative stress both in the lipid phase of biological membranes and in an aqueous environment. NAC is proposed to treat ocular disorders which have the component of oxidative stress in their genesis (cataracts, glaucoma, retinal degeneration, corneal disorders, ocular inflammation, complications of diabetes mellitus, systemic diseases).

PMID: 8894306 [PubMed—indexed for MEDLINE]

Clin Chim Acta. 1996 Oct 15;254(1):1-21. Related Articles, Links Erratum in: Clin Chim Acta 1997 Mar 18;259(1-2): 199-201.

N alpha-acetylcarnosine is a prodrug of L-carnosine in ophthalmic application as antioxidant.

Babizhayev MA, Yermakova VN, Sakina NL, Evstigneeva RR Rozhkova EA, Zheltukhina GA

Resources for Your 10 Step™ Action Plan

Call the help line, shown at the front of the book for help in locating sources.

Nutrient

MaxiFocus Spray (not tablets or capsules)

Contains: Lutein, Zeaxanthin and 22 natural nutrients recommended for eye health.

Liquid Vitamins and Minerals

Contains: Every essential vitamin and minerals in liquid form

Taurine Spray

Contains: Taurine, an amino acid for the eyes and brain

Astaxanthin

Antioxidant formula, many times more powerful than Vitamin E

MSM+Silver water drops

Contains: Colloidal Silver, Sterilised water, methyl sulfonyl methane, ionic Zinc

HealthPoint Microcurrent stimulator

All the power of acupuncture, without needles

Essential Fatty Acids

Can be Hemp Oi for vegetarians or any fish oil complex with 480mg DHA and 720mg EPA per serving

OxySorb

Contains: Seaweed extract to improve oxygenation

Sprouted Wheat Bread

Contains: 100% Organic sprouted wheat grains and filtered water.

R-Alpha Lipoic Acid

Contains: 100mg Alpha Lipoic Acid

Digestive Enzymes

Contains: full spectrum of plant (not animal) digestive enzymes

Lycopene

Contains: 100mg of Lycopene and other nutrients

Whole body and Colon Cleanse

Contains: a 30 day supply of body and colon cleanse

Serrapeptase

Contains: an enzyme for arterial diseases and inflammation

Curcumin98

Promotes glutathione to help prevent cataracts (and much more)

Pancreas Plus

Contains: Gymnema Sylvestre, MSM, Chromium, Vanadium, Boron and Niacin

Probiotic14

Contains 14 strains of friendly bacteria for the digestive system

Bilberry/Gingko Formula

Contains: Gingko and Bilberry for circulation, stroke prevention and to protect against leaky veins.

Vitamin E

Contains: Alpha Tocopheryl Acetate 1,000IU per capsule

Can-C drops

Contains: N-Acetyl carnosine for the control of cataracts

Revision Herbal Formula

Contains: a herbal formula to support the eyes and the liver

Vision Tone Herbal Formula

Contains: a herbal formula to strengthen the eyes

Viva Eye Drops

For dry eyes

Thera Tears

For severe dry eye conditions

More Books to read (when your eyesight returns)

The Miracle Enzyme is Serrapeptase	Robert Redfern
MicroCurrent Stimulation: Miracle Eye Cure (USA)	Edward C. Kondrot MD
The Bates Method (UK)	Dr Peter Mansfield
Racketeering In Medicine (USA)	James P. Carter MD
What Doctors Don't Tell You (UK)	Lynne McTaggart
What Doctors Wont Tell You (USA)	Jane Heimlich
The Story Of Medicine (UK)	Dr. Vernon Coleman
Betrayal Of Trust	Dr. Vernon Coleman
The Glucose Revolution	Dr. Anthony Leeds
Your Body Cries For Water	Dr. Fereydoon Batmanghelid

Any Recipe books for wheat- and sugar-free living.

Useful Websites

www.Eyesight.nu

www.DoveHealth.com

www.CurcuminHealth.info

www.Serrapeptase.info

www.ReallyHealthyFoods.com

www.GoodHealthNews.tv

See the website **www.eyesight.nu** for more help, or call the help line, shown at the front of the book, with your specific questions.